HEATHEN

RICHARD BAUD

WESTBOW
PRESS®
A DIVISION OF THOMAS NELSON
& ZONDERVAN

WestBow Press books may be ordered through booksellers or by contacting:

WestBow Press
A Division of Thomas Nelson & Zondervan
1663 Liberty Drive
Bloomington, IN 47403
www.westbowpress.com
844-714-3454

All Scripture quotations are taken from the King James Version, public domain.

ISBN: 979-8-3850-3005-7 (sc)
ISBN: 979-8-3850-3006-4 (e)

Library of Congress Control Number: 2024915100

Print information available on the last page.

WestBow Press rev. date: 08/05/2024

CONTENTS

INTRODUCTION

After leaving the working world, I am deciding what to do with the years I have left. I am 60 years old, my mother died at 74, my biological father died at 74. So, I figure that I have some time left on this earth. What do I do with this precious time? I will spend as much time as possible with my family, especially my grandchildren.

I have a lot of hard-earned experience over my 60 years. And I would like to share that hard earned experience with my community. Exactly how to do this I am not sure, but as a Christian I look for God to lead me.

As I reflect on my past and contemplate my future. I am constantly being brought back to two things. First, how God has brought me to the point he has in life. Second, how I need to share this journey with others.

So, before I go forward in life, I will follow God's gentle nudge. And thru this book explain what God has done for me.

I am not a professional author, but I will do my best to tell my story from my perspective.

The title of this book is heathen as you will discover in Chapter 1. Me and my siblings were called this name by some good Christian kids in my hometown when I was young.

This book is dedicated to my mother Mavis Grieves. Mom you were a mighty force in my life and I look forward to seeing you in Heaven.

MY BEGINNINGS

My mother had been pregnant when she divorced my biological father when I was two years old. My mom made the choice to give that child up for adoption. She arranged for her brother and his wife to adopt him. This couple could not have kids and they were in a good situation to take care of him.

The earliest I can remember, my mom was with the man that would become her third husband, James F. Grieves. Jim was 20 years older than my mom and had lost his left arm in an electrical accident. So, the family that I remember growing up with consisted of Jim, my stepfather, Mom, four children from mom's first marriage with Bill Ruffner, and two boys and two girls. This part of my family had the oldest children. Two children from my mom's second marriage to my biological father James Paul Baud. I am the oldest, my little brother Tom followed me by 17 months. The child that was adopted would make three boys from my mom and biological father. Note: I knew nothing about my adopted-out brother until I turned 18 years old. (Mom told each of us kids on our 18th birthday.) So, while growing up I thought it was me and Tom only, from my mom and biological father. Two children from my mom's third marriage to James F. Grieves. Both of their children were girls, one born in 1967 and one born in 1968. These two girls were very special to my stepdad as he was 50 years old when they arrived on the scene. So, that was my family Mom, Jim (stepdad), four Ruffner children, two Baud children, two Grieves children. My immediate family had a total of ten people. This was the family that I remember and was raised with.

Where we lived: My family moved around a lot when I was very young. From these years I have no memory but we lived in places all over Crawford County Illinois. Including one house that had a house fire.

Then at some point we relocated to the Chicago, Illinois area. We lived in Chicago Heights, Illinois, Hammond, Indiana and Griffith, Indiana. I recall a few things from this time period. First, it was very cold in this area. Second, I wore a parka to my school that helped with the cold. Third, some of my siblings went to the same school (I could see them during recess.) Fourth, we went to school via taxicab, not sure how or why. Fifth, in the winter of 1967 in January we had 23 inches of snow. That shut down a lot of that area. My stepdad was stuck in the part of town he worked in for three days before he could return home. Sixth, our next-door neighbor was stabbed to death, we moved back to Crawford County after that. One of our houses was in the country outside of Oblong, Illinois. At this place at least for a time we had no running water. So, my stepdad would take trash cans over to my Aunt Louellen's house and fill them up so we could have water. We lived next to a river that flooded a lot. When this happened, the school bus could not get to our house. So we missed school those days. One vivid memory of mine was of a terrified cow, floating down the swollen river this scared me half to death.

We moved to town in Oblong, Illinois. This was a town that had a population of under 2,000 people. We moved into a house on Cross Street. This was a big two-story house. It was old but had lots of room, which we needed with 10 people living there. My stepdad worked very hard to fix it up including tearing down and replacing entire walls. My stepdad could do electrical work, plumbing, carpentry, and of course painting. This was my favorite house growing up. While living at this house, we had one week where temperatures did not get over zero degrees day or night. Is stopped everyone, car batteries died, and you had to heat the dip stick on your car to keep it from freezing. This house burned to the ground. Apparently, the furnace caught on fire and consumed the whole house. The day I returned to school I overheard my teacher say that we probably burned down the house for insurance money. I didn't think so because my stepdad worked so hard to fix up that house. And we lost everything including old photos and our Christmas presents that were hidden in the house. When the house burned down, we temporally moved into the local motel, the Arvin Motel. (The insurance company put us up as part of the insurance policy.) That was a weird couple of weeks with so many people living in a motel. Then we moved into a very small house, in a very small town of Stoy, Illinois. Basically just a few houses. There was a field across the street from our house where me and my siblings and other kids would play football and other games. At this house me and my brothers tried to burn some coal that was in the shed, nearly burning down the shed. We later moved in a very old run-down house right across from the railroad tracks and a big grain storage silo facility. That house had not been painted in years and looked very bad. The room that I stayed in had a big enough hole in it that I could stick my hand outside the wall, making it quite cold in the Illinois winter. At this house me and brothers found unspent rifle shells and decided it would be neat to explode the shells. We put them on a brick and hit them with a hammer. That made a very loud noise as they exploded. Miraculously no one was hurt. We moved to 404 North Division Street. My parents bought a double wide trailer and moved it onto the property. My stepdad built the septic tank drain system himself. We lived in this double wide trailer longer than any other place that I can remember. At some point we moved to Crossville, Illinois another small town. My mom and stepdad bought an old fashion restaurant in that town. We moved into an odd house that was referred to as The Apple House. Apparently, apples were sold there at some point. At the restaurant all of us kids worked there, washing dishes, cleaning floors, waiting tables, etc. When the high school had home games some of us would go to the game. And if we won the game we would race home and inform our parents of the win, that would be a very busy night at the restaurant. When the restaurant started doing badly, we moved to an old house in the country outside Crossville. It was at this house that the repo man showed up and wanted to take my stepdads station wagon. (Our only vehicle.) My stepdad was able to avoid it but it was a scary day for a little kid. Later another repo guy came and picked up some of our furniture and appliances. After a few months the restaurant was dealt a death blow with a $400 electric bill and closed. When the restaurant failed, we moved back to Oblong. Back to the same trailer at 404 North Division Street. We lived in this trailer until the day I left home at 18 years old. While at this trailer, we had another fire. My stepdad was trying to thaw out frozen pipes by using a blow torch. The insulation caught fire and destroyed part of the trailer. Once again we lost hidden Christmas presents.

We were very poor the entire time we were growing up. I don't want to over state how poor we were, but it did make an impact on my early life, so I will give you a few examples. One day my stepdad had run out of cigarettes and had no money to buy more, me and my brothers were headed to the local lake to go fishing, my stepdad asked us to sell some of the worms to other fishers at the lake to raise money for his cigarettes. We did as told and raised enough money to buy a pack of cigarettes. We did the same thing one day that mom had no money and needed butter for supper. One day I was in grade school and was wearing worn out tennis shoes to physical education class. The physical education teacher said I could not be on the gym with shoes in that condition. We had no money to buy new shoes, so I was kept home from school the next day. That was a Friday, Mom was somehow able to buy me a pair of tennis shoes that weekend. One of the most embarrassing things about being poor was at lunch time at the school cafeteria, one of the teachers would announce "kids that get free lunch line up here." They separated those who got government help with lunch. "Probably for reporting purposes." But we all felt like second class citizens.

One girl passing by our house threw rocks at my dog King, King was a German Shepard who was able to break his chain and chase the girl and bit her on the foot. Later that day an officer came to our house and told my mom and stepdad that we could either pay a fine or get rid of the dog. We had no money, so my dog King was taken away from me. This was one of the worst memories of my life. I loved that dog. It was not fair because the girl had thrown rocks at him.

My stepdad had made it clear that we would not take welfare. And he did not until he lost his job and had no choice. Back then it wasn't much but it did give us, free school lunches, food stamps, big blocks of cheese.

The big blocks of cheese were part of the federal government subsidy of dairy farmers, to keep the prices up for dairy farmers. The government would take the excess cheese that was produced and give that excess cheese to poor families. Once a month we would go to a distribution point and prove our income was low enough, then we would receive some of that cheese.

When I was in seventh grade, we were told to study The Declaration of Independence, then all seventh graders would be tested on it. When they graded the test, I got one of the highest scores in my class. Which entitled me and the other top scorers to be ushers at the graduation of the eighth graders. So all was set and I was prepared to do it, then I was told that we had to wear a suit for boys and a dress for girls. Well, I did not own a suit. My parents did not have enough money for a suit for me so I told my teacher that I did not have a suit and could not do it. I left this experience with a thought that doing good in school was not for me and my efforts in school went down.

One afternoon my siblings and I were playing in the front yard when a nice-looking station wagon drove by loaded with a family of good Christians dressed up for church, they were headed home after church. All of a sudden, a couple of the children rolled down their window and shouted, "Look at the heathens." I heard the words but did not really understand them. I'd heard that word before. I'd watched many westerns on tv and that is a word that the white people would call the Indians. Me and my siblings shrugged it off, but I thought about that incident over the years with sadness, no one likes to be called names. Near Christmas one year my Uncle Lawrence died in a fire in my aunt's trailer. This of course is awful, but it was made worse by the circumstances. You see Uncle Lawrence was unique. He had been put in a mental institution. He apparently was not mentally ill, but it was convenient for his parents to put him there, so they did. Uncle Lawrence spent many years in that mental institution with folks who were truly mentally ill, causing him to be different. He had learned how to survive in an institution with very rigid rules. One of these rules was that he could not leave his bedroom until he was fully dressed. My aunt (his half-sister) took him out of the institution after he was a middle-aged man and made him part of her family. Uncle Lawrence was different but adjusted well. He could not drive so he would ride a bicycle everywhere. You would see him a lot of places around town, riding his bike, happy as could be. Uncle Lawrence wore that bike out and my aunt decided to surprise him with a new bike for Christmas. To keep it a surprise she could not keep the bike under the Christmas tree. Instead, she had a Christmas card on the Christmas tree with a note inside telling Uncle Lawrence about the bike. This was to be opened Christmas Day. Uncle Lawrence kept looking for a bike under the Christmas tree but of course there never was a bike under the Christmas tree, that would have ruined the big surprise. Tragically before Christmas that year my aunts trailer caught on fire. Everyone else was safe but Uncle Lawrence, who was trained at the mental institution never to leave your bedroom unless fully dressed, was overcome with smoke as he tried to hurry up and get dressed. He died that day.

Some of the best memories I have growing up was fishing at the community lake in Oblong, Illinois. Me and my brothers and sisters would go there a lot. It was a small lake, but it was stocked well, and it was a great place to spend a summer day. We would find the worms in our yard after a big rain. So fishing was free and even our family could afford that. And mom fried the fish we caught, so it must have helped her with her task of making her food budget stretch to feed all 10 of us. We lived on the other side of town, so it was quite a long walk, but we never minded, the trip there and back was tiring but we managed it.

One of our local citizens, Tom Cook owned and operated a restaurant a few blocks from downtown Oblong and close to the high school. This business was always busy and a gathering place for lots of people. Me and my little brother Tom spent a ton of time there. As soon as we were old enough, we would mow neighbors' yards and gain enough money to go to Tom Cooks. Tom Cooks was across town from where we lived so we would walk to get there. Sometimes we would have enough money to get a burger for lunch, sometimes not. But every time we went there, we would play the pin ball machine. The cost to play was 10 cents per game, and if you were good enough at it you could get a high enough score to win a free game. Well, after playing the same game for years, you get good at it and me and my little brother could play for hours for a couple of dimes. We would spend half the day there some days.

My aunt at some point was married to a farmer and me and my

siblings would take turns spending time helping my aunt and uncle out on the farm, learning how to take care of the animals and taking care of the farm. I remember during the winters it would be so cold that the lake would freeze and my uncle would have to break up the ice for the livestock to drink.

Years later my aunt was married to a man name Russ. I learned how to hunt from this guy. We would spend hours hunting squirrels and rabbits. I really liked to hunt and when I stayed at their house I would hunt by myself, and got really good at shooting squirrels in the head with a 22 inch rifle. Once I fell asleep hunting squirrels, I woke up to find a squirrel on my rifle barrel looking straight at me, probably laughing and taunting me.

Me and my little brother's biological father was rarely around. My grandmother on my biological father's side, Dorothy Skidmore, and my uncle Larry Baud who is my biological father's brother, did what they could to fill in the gap that our absentee father left. They would take us to see other family members on my father's side and keep us involved in the greater Baud family. Me and my younger brother would spend part of the summer with Uncle Larry and his family. These were fun times. Uncle Larry was a great example of how to prioritize your children and have a good time with your family.

My stepdad would paint houses and businesses to earn money, he seemed to enjoy that line of work better than his other job over the years at machine shops and factories. One summer he took me with him to help paint a country church. This was hard work, but it was very fulfilling, and my stepdad gave me $20 for helping him, a big deal in my life.

Growing up my family was very poor, and we were on the low end of the social and economic ladder. I was never motivated to do good at school, the deck was always stacked against me, and the future did not seem very promising.

Then on November 1, 1977, I got a new job at a retailer in Robinson, Illinois named Pamida. This was just a temporary job, I was hired as Christmas help and would do whatever was needed, including stocking shelves, cleaning restrooms, sweeping floors, running cash register. Whatever was needed. At first, I was timid and apprehensive, but I learned how to do stuff and discovered all you had to do to succeed there was to show up on time and to work hard. I took to this line of work with ease and found myself (for the first time in my life). Unlike school equal to everyone else that worked there. Living the American dream for me started here. I was able to show up, work hard and excel at what I was doing. Nothing else mattered to my bosses except what work I did. So, I put every ounce of effort into this job and was able to move up in that store quickly. I learned work is an awesome way to be proud of yourself and your accomplishments.

RICHARD BAUD

CHAPTER 2

GOING DOWN THE
WRONG PATH

So, as many people do, I had some trouble going from a child to an adult. My teenage years were made more difficult for me because of a couple of factors. First, my older brothers stayed in trouble and were not a positive influence on me. I will give you a few examples: At the school cafeteria if you wanted an individual box of milk for lunch you were supposed to drop a nickel in a basket and pick up your milk as you headed to the lunch tables. My two older brothers would drop in a nickel and take out a quarter.

When our high school had a hometown game my oldest brother would always volunteer to take money for admission to the game. Whenever no one was looking he would pocket as much money as he could.

My older brothers would mow yards to pick up spending money. You did not get rich mowing yards, but it was a reliable source of funds when your parents could not afford anything except the very basics. So, one day one of the people they mowed yards for, came to the door of our house with a police officer complaining that my older brothers had changed the amount on the check that she had gave them.

This kind of behavior would continue and escalate to the point where they were both all-out criminals and they both stayed in and out of jail and prison for my entire teenage years. And continuing many years afterwards.

The second major driving factor driving me down the wrong path was my taste for alcohol. I give my biological father the credit for setting an awful example for me and my little brother when it comes to alcohol consumption. According to my mom he became addicted to wine when he was in the military stationed in France. So, as I was headed for the dangerous teenage years, he was constantly in the local newspaper for his DUI arrest. So, I jumped head long into every irresponsible situation that I could think about getting into. I will start with some of the mischief that me and my brothers were involved in. Halloween time was a time for us to be bad. When we would do the normal toilet papering trees of random neighbors and mean teachers. We would also pile leaves in the middle of the street and light them on fire. We would put a safety pin strategically placed under the hood to make the horn blow, if it continued the battery died or someone removed the safety pin. In the winter we would roll up an ice ball made of snow and ice and hit cars with them as they drove by. We would throw them from the alley and run before the car could stop and the driver could get out.

Now I will tell about some of what I did during my high school years. I guess I started drinking around age 14. It came by me very naturally. During shop class me and some of my friends would replace Pepsi with Vodka or Whiskey and drink it during class. The shop teacher was very old and never caught us. In my Junior year I had a class that was not taught at my school in Oblong. I had to commute everyday to neighboring Robinson, Illinois, where they taught that specific class. On the way to class and on the way home, me and some of my classmates would race each other the nine miles going speeds up to 100 miles an hour. A few miles from Robinson there was an S curve, and we would pass each other going thru the S curve playing a very dangerous game of chicken.

Many nights driving home I was so drunk that by the time I got home I could not remember the drive home. I hung out with many other kids not motivated to excel in addition to heavy drinking we would smoke marijuana. We would smoke it during lunch hour and on the way home from school. During assembly you would see a smoke cloud coming from the top bleachers, where we would sit and smoke pot not sure how we were never noticed.

I went to a party with one of my friends in Palestine, Illinois that was supplied with more serious drugs including pills. There was a game with lots of different pills were put in a basket. You picked one and took it and waited to see what it would do to you.

As I headed for destruction four situations happened that any one of which could have ended up with me being killed or in serious trouble. Situation No. 1: When I was 15 years old, my older brother (he was three years older than me) invited me to a night of drinking. We ended up going to his wife's parents' home. His wife was 18 years old, she was pregnant and had left him and moved back to her parents' home. My brother had wanted to convince her to take him back. I stayed in the car while he went to talk to his separated wife. In about five minutes I heard yelling and saw a man holding a shot gun chasing my brother who was running to the car where I was and was being shot at while he was running. I thought two things: First, this seems like an ignorant mistake hanging out with my ignorant brother. Second, I better get out of the line of fire. So I started up the car, my brother caught up with me and his car and we took off. This is the first time I was rescued from a serious incident by a God I did not know.

Situation No. 2: A year later on my sixteenth birthday, I was driving my car with my younger brother riding with me. I was driving my car down a black top road and as the road turned into a gravel road, I meant to slow down but hit the gas pedal by mistake. The car started sliding and went off the road into a ditch and took out a fence row. My brother started yelling that he was bleeding and in reality, the windshield had rust from the fence on it and my brother thought it was blood. We had survived this wreck uninjured. This is the second time I was rescued by a God I did not know.

Situation No. 3: Within the next few months I made the worst mistake I had ever made. When one of my friends invited me to a keg party on a nearby farm. I arrived late in the afternoon and did like everyone else, got drunk. Now that is bad enough, but it got a lot worse. The keg party was near a lake, and everyone was swinging from a very large swing and swinging over the lake and jumping into the lake. This looked like a lot of fun, everyone else was doing it so I thought I would do it also. As I was half over the lake, I remembered that I could not swim. I sank like a rock. Drunk and unable to swim I started thrashing around in the water. After a few minutes (it seemed like a month) one of my friends saw me struggling and jumped into the lake to help. I remember feeling very helpless and how great it was to breath air again. This was the third time I was rescued from a serious incident by a God I did not know.

Near Halloween I was driving my car and my younger brother was riding with me. We were cruising our small town of Oblong, Illinois and in a very old and very big Buick (all of a sudden, some car started following us). Apparently, a car that looked like mine was involved in stealing two bikes from a neighborhood we were driving thru. And in the car that was following us was two men that was part of a civil patrol. These men were helping to keep our streets safe and were in an unmarked vehicle. As they neared my car they put on their flashing lights. I made a snap decision to evade these guys. It started as a slow speed chase with only that car following us. As the chase progressed, I kept going faster and going thru alleys and side roads and parking lots. Eventually police cars joined the chase, and it was turning into a wild situation. I don't know how fast I went but it was very dangerous, as I was headed out of town some police cars cut in front of me and blocked my way out. As the police had their guns pulled and headed to my car, I was able to make up a quick story. The police officer told me to get out of the car and asked me what I was doing. I told the officer that the unmarked car started following me and I thought the men inside had a rifle. I told the officer I was thinking they were criminals and that is why I took off. Somehow the police believed me and let me go. This was a new low for me, I had endangered my life and my little brother's life. This was the fourth time I was rescued from a serious incident by a God I did not know. Alcohol, marijuana, and poor decisions had come together to really mess me up and any kind of future I might have. But God had plans for me and would slowly move me to where he wanted me.

CHAPTER 3

GOD TAKES CONTROL

I n chapters one and two of this book I explain how my childhood unfolded and gave various examples of how God had looked out for me when I was growing up. This chapter will show how God guided me from my early adult years to where I am now.

I worked at Pamida from age 16 to age 19. I had found my niche in life in retail, and I was able to move from stock boy to group manager in those three years. Then on December 30, 1980, I went to work at Walmart as a management trainee. Walmart really did not pay me much more than I made at Pamida but I had noticed that whenever Walmart moved into a town lots of other places closed. So I decided to jump over to Walmart before the same thing happened to my Pamida.

I worked my way from management trainee to Assistant Manager then finally after four and a half years I was promoted to Store Manager of the Walmart in Russellville, Kentucky. I now know that this was part of God's plan for me and was the beginning of my search for peace and happiness. I was totally alone in Kentucky. I knew no one. I was lonelier there than I had ever been in my life. I was a young man, 24 years old put in a position where I knew that I would have to rely on myself to begin a new life. I had just been named manager of my first store, so I decided to put everything into my work. I spent every waking hour trying to make myself and my store a success. I learned a lot the first six months about being a store manager and about myself. I learned that I could do whatever I had to do. It is amazing that when you have no other choice than to succeed what you can push yourself to do. As I said earlier this was the loneliest times of my life. For even though I spent all my time at work, when I came home to my one room studio apartment, I had to face me, myself, for I had no one else. I was searching for the reason I was there. Nothing else made any sense. I never really had anyone very close to me to talk to, so I tried to work these things out for myself (guess what). I never figured out anything. At the time I couldn't even tell you why I was alive or what life was all about.

As I write this book in 2021 I have found God or really God found me, but in 1985 I did not know God. Growing up we were a family that did not talk about God and went to church only a handful of times when my stepdad was painting that church. I remember a couple of times when my stepdad slammed the door in the face of people who came from the local church to tell us about Jesus. I thank God that my stepdad accepted the Lord on his death bed when he died of cancer on February 18, 1980, which was my youngest sister's 12th birthday.

While I was in the darkest period of my life there was someone who was asking God to send her a Godly man. This person was Ramona. Who would one day become my wife. I previously said Ramona had been praying for a Godly man. At the time we met I was not a Godly man. I think I was a normal person who was doing the best that I could without God. It was after Ramona and I had married that I began to feel that I had been sent to Russellville, Kentucky for a reason. After I married Ramona, I began to see how differently she had been raised. Her parents were Christians and had brought up their children in church. What a difference that makes!!!!!!!! I could see that their family was very close and were grounded in their faith. Soon after we were married Ramona and I began going to some different churches in the Russellville area, something I was not used to. Over the next several years I began to make a new life with Ramona. We had two boys already between us Richard Baud, Jr. and Joshua Owen Thomas. And soon we had children of our own. Samuel Baud born 9-17-87 and Katie Baud born 12-5-89. I had been given bigger Walmart stores to manage and we had moved several times. Each time we moved we went to new churches. I seemed to fit in alright at each of these churches. I listened to the music and to the preacher and left the same as I came in, unsaved. We didn't go to church regularly. Just every once in a while.

I don't know what would bring us to church. Ramona would request that we go sometimes, and it just seemed to me like we needed to go on occasion. I remember saying to people that it really doesn't matter if you go to church. God is everywhere and all you have to do is be a good person and you will be fine.

After several years in the Kentucky, Tennessee area we moved to Virginia. After a short time in Richmond, Virginia and Alexandria, Virginia we ended up in Manassas, Virginia. Like all other places we had lived we tried local churches and would go to worship service on Sunday morning and feel like we had done our part. We had gone to church and had listened to the preacher and felt good when we left church. We still only went to church when we felt like it, very sporadically.

It was the year 1995, late in September when the world changed for my family. We had lived in Virginia a little more than four years. As we headed west of our home in Manassas, Virginia, we were out on a road trip to see the beauty of the mountains, that we could only barely see from home. It was a fall day, the leaves were beginning to turn colors and the scenery was amazing as we passed a church that stood tall on a hill. Samuel who was eight years old pointed to the church and asked, "Daddy what does that T stand for?" I looked over at my wife Ramona as she looked at me. Ramona explained to Samuel that the T stood for the cross that Jesus had died on. I cannot explain the horrible feelings that both me and Ramona felt at that very moment. I thought how can my eight years old son not know about Jesus. Then I realized that I really did not either.

Well, I knew that something was missing in my life and that little question that Samuel raised shook my world. Ramona and I decided to go and visit that church (Battlefield Baptist Church) where Samuel had asked that important question, "Daddy what does that T stand for."

So, we started going to Battlefield Baptist Church. We both liked the church; something was different about it to me. It seemed more serious. More real and of course there was the preacher, Karl Skinner. How do I describe this man? He was a man about fifty years old, rather short, nearly bald and kind of chunky. I had never ever heard someone preach like he did. He said the words like he actually meant and believed them. He was animated, he jumped up and down, he was positive and enthusiastic. WOW!!!! We went to this church every Sunday for worship service. The entire family went, sometimes willingly and sometimes not so willingly, but we all went and soon we started talking about God. Samuel and the rest of us learned about Jesus and what that T stands for. It became normal to go to church.

Every week I understood more about the church and what it is all about. Every week during the invitation our pastor Karl Skinner pleaded with those who didn't know Jesus to accept his free gift of salvation. At first, I thought it was a waste of time. How could just going up to the front of the church and talking to the preacher do anything. Well, as the weeks went by I began to understand, because as the preacher was talking, I began to feel something inside of me telling me that I was lost and needed the Lord. Each Sunday the tug on my heart became stronger and stronger. I realized that it was just a matter of time before I would have to make a decision. But every Sunday I would resist and come up with reasons in my head why it shouldn't be this week. Then while I was doing my job working at Walmart in the middle of the Christmas season it happened. Lennette Hutt, my domestics department manager said, "here Richard read this poem, it is really good." This is the poem I read that day.

TWAS THE NIGHT BEFORE
JESUS CAME

Twas the night before Jesus came and all through the house,
Not a creature was praying, not one in the house.
Their Bibles were lain on the shelf without care,
In hopes that Jesus would not come there.

The children were dressing to crawl into bed,
Not once ever kneeling or bowing a head.
And Mom in the rocker with Baby on her lap,
Was watching the Late Show while I took a nap.

When out of the East there arose such a clatter,
I sprang to my feet to see what was the matter.
Away to the window I flew like a flash!
Tore open the shutters and threw up the sash!

When what to my wondering eyes should appear,
But angels proclaiming that Jesus was here!
With a light like the sun sending forth a bright ray,
I knew in a moment this must be the day.

The light of his face made me cover my heard,
It was Jesus returning just like he said.
And though I possessed worldly wisdom and wealth,
I cried when I saw him in spite of myself.

In The Book of Life which he held in his hand,
Was written the name of every saved man.
He spoke not a word as he searched for my name,
When he said "It's not here." My head hung in shame.

The people whose names had been written with love,
He gathered to take to his Father above.
With those who were ready he arose without a sound,
While all the rest were left standing around.

I fell to my knees, but it was too late,
I had waited too long and thus sealed my fate.
I stood and I cried as they arose out of sight,
Oh, if only I had been ready tonight!

In the words of this poem the meaning is clear,
The coming of Jesus is drawing near.
There's only one life and when comes the last call,
We'll find that the Bible was true after all!

I read this poem and I was immediately overpowered with the Holy Spirit telling me to quit stalling and to accept the offer of salvation. I had no choice, I made the decision to be saved that coming Sunday, Sunday 12-15-96 came, I announced that morning before church that I made the decision and would go down the aisle. I did this in advance to set an example for my children. When we got to church I could not tell you what Pastor Skinner's message was. I could only think about getting down the aisle and getting saved. When the invitation came, I went down the aisle and accepted the Lord Jesus Christ as my personal Lord and Savior. The same day 12-15-96 I was baptized. Since that day I have had an inner peace that I never knew that I could ever have. That day 12-15-96 I gave up drinking alcohol. No longer needing it to get by in life. Since 12-15-96 I know without any doubt that when I die, I will go to heaven. I hope to live my life in a way that will glorify the Lord.

From the second the Lord saved me I've had a heavy burden to see my family saved. All of my family, my own children and my extended family. As I have said earlier, I had not grown up in a church and I was only now really learning about what it meant to be a Christian. So I knew that I needed to get to church and learn all that I needed to learn to be a good Christian and to help lead my family to Christ. So we started to expand the time we dedicated to church. We had only been going to Sunday a.m. worship so I told my family that we would start going to Sunday evening service. They didn't like it but we started going each week, Sunday a.m. and Sunday p.m. I thought that we should start going to Sunday School, this was not popular at our house, but we did it anyway. Sunday School was great, it helped teach me and my children the basics of the Bible and where we fit in God's plans. Well the last shoe dropped, I insisted that we go to church on Wednesday night for prayer service. No one was happy. My family fought this every Wednesday until they finally gave in.

So within a few months there we were going from a family who only went to church occasionally to a family who went to church every time the doors were open, praise God. This was truly a miracle in my family.

It was only a few months after I was saved that my youngest son Samuel made the decision the accept the Lord as his Savior. This was a wonderful day, how great is it to know that your child is going to heaven, Samuel was saved on 2-2-1997.

Shortly after that my only daughter, Katherine said she wanted to be saved. She understood what it meant, she was still a young girl age 7, but she was ready to be saved and went down the aisle on 4-6-1997.

My other son Josh had been saved a couple of years earlier as he had gone to a Christian school when he was younger. So, the time was at hand to reach out to my older son Richard Baud, Jr. As he was growing up, I didn't have God so I couldn't teach him about God, but this changed 12-15-1996. So I set out to make up for lost time. I began to discuss God and my experiences with Richard, Jr. Every time I seen him and every time I talked to him. During the summer of 1997 I spent a week with Richard, Jr. trying to teach him what I now knew. All my efforts were met with curiosity but not with acceptance, but I kept trying. I knew it was not me, but God who could save Richard, Jr. So I prayed every day that Richard, Jr. would accept the Lord. My focus was on my last unsaved child, but it was apparent that it would take time, so I began to reach out to my extended family. This has been tough. As you now know my family was not a church going family, and what I was saying probably sounding incomprehensible to my extended family. But I have a passion to see every member of my family saved. So I will do whatever I can to make this happen. I realize only God can save a person, but the Bible teaches that we have the power to pray to God and God promises to answer our prayers. So I call out the names of my extended family to God, and I ask him to save them in the name of Jesus Christ. In May 1998 we moved to Columbia, Tn. And after trying out every Baptist church in town at least once some twice we decided to join Northside Baptist Church. I will tell you more about Northside Baptist Church in a future chapter.

After we had been at Northside Baptist Church, I was asked by pastor John Rushing to give my testimony and discuss it in relation to stewardship month. It came to me that this testimony might be helpful in witnessing to my extended family. So I made up a list of my extended family and sent each a copy of my testimony on stewardship on 3-1-2000. This is a copy of that letter.

Dear Family Members:

Recently I was asked to speak to my church about stewardship. This got me to thinking that I should also share my story with my family. So that is what this letter is about.

Growing up I remember our family going to church a few times, but we were not a family which discussed God or regularly attended church.

When I met Ramona she was from a family which went to church every week so we started to try out different churches every town we moved to.

At these churches I was able to learn about religion but I have to tell you that it was only words I was hearing.

That all changed one day in December 1996, when one of my department managers at Wal-Mart gave me a poem to read. This poem is called "Twas The Night Before Jesus Came." (See poem attached)

As I read this poem I was crushed, for the first time I realized that I was not going to heaven and I was never going to see Jesus, and as a result of my failure my children would be destined for the same future. I realized that Hell was real and that I had decisions to make.

For the next couple of days Jesus worked on me. I felt his presence and I made the decision to accept him as my personal savior.

That Sunday 12-15-96, after the preacher was finished with his sermon, I walked down the aisle and accepted Jesus as my personal savior. The preacher read some Bible versus. Romans Chapter 3 verse 23, chapter 6 verse 23, chapter 5 verse 8, chapter 10 verse 9-10, and chapter 10 verse 13. Then I prayed this prayer, "Jesus I know I am a sinner, please forgive me of my sins. I am asking you to come in to my life and save me." Immediately I knew that Jesus had made good on his promises and that I was saved. I have felt differently ever since then. I now have a peace in my life that I never knew before. I know that if I die today, I will go to heaven and spend eternity with Jesus.

TWAS THE NIGHT BEFORE
JESUS CAME

Twas the night before Jesus came and all through the house,
Not a creature was praying, not one in the house.
Their Bibles were lain on the shelf without care,
In hopes that Jesus would not come there.

The children were dressing to crawl into bed,
Not once ever kneeling or bowing a head.
And Mom in the rocker with Baby on her lap,
Was watching the Late Show while I took a nap.

When out of the East there arose such a clatter,
I sprang to my feet to see what was the matter.
Away to the window I flew like a flash!
Tore open the shutters and threw up the sash!

When what to my wondering eyes should appear,
But angels proclaiming that Jesus was here!
With a light like the sun sending forth a bright ray,
I knew in a moment this must be the day.

The light of his face made me cover my heard,
It was Jesus returning just like he said.
And though I possessed worldly wisdom and wealth,
I cried when I saw him in spite of myself.

In The Book of Life which he held in his hand,
Was written the name of every saved man.
He spoke not a word as he searched for my name,
When he said "It's not here." My head hung in shame.

The people whose names had been written with love,
He gathered to take to his Father above.
With those who were ready he arose without a sound,
While all the rest were left standing around.

I fell to my knees, but it was too late,
I had waited too long and thus sealed my fate.
I stood and I cried as they arose out of sight,
Oh, if only I had been ready tonight!

In the words of this poem the meaning is clear,
The coming of Jesus is drawing near.
There's only one life and when comes the last call,
We'll find that the Bible was true after all!

Since I was saved, Samuel, Katie, and Richard Jr. have all accepted Jesus and I know where they will spend eternity. I do not know how anyone who does not have this peace can sleep at night.

The day Jesus came into my life the holy spirit took up residence in me and I started hearing God speak thru the preacher.

The Sunday after I was saved our pastor preached from Malachi 3 Versus 7-11. I wanted to be obedient to God's command so I started to tithe 10% of my pay. The next Sunday our pastor said he needed to clarify that the 10% needed to come off the top. He said that the taxes, social security, etc. was between us and the government. God wants us to give him the 1st 10% and to do it cheerfully.

I thought to myself what is he going to ask for next Sunday, but I wanted to do what God commanded so I started tithing 10% off the top. I continued to tithe and to go to church and learned more about God's word including his promises such as Luke 6 verse 38. The pastor said we could never out give God.

After we started tithing things changed for my family, things we had wanted to do (but had always had stumbling blocks put up in our way) finally started happening.

I'll give you a few examples: (1) We were in Virginia and wanted to move back closer to home, but after trying several times to transfer with Wal-Mart we basically gave up on moving back. (2) So we decided we would stay in Virginia. We loved our church and our pastor. We decided to buy a house in 1999. In March of 1998 our landlords decided to move back to their house, and we had 60 days to move out. If you are ever in that position you do not feel like you are about to be blest. So we figured we would just go ahead and buy a house a little earlier than we planned on.

It sounded like a good plan except nothing worked out. There was not much housing available in the first place, and Samuel had school and neighbor friends and wanted to go to the same school they did which limited our area to find a house. Time was moving on and we were faced with a date to move out. So we did what we should have done first, we prayed and asked God to lead us and we agreed to follow God's will.

I don't remember exactly why I did it but I looked at the stores

Wal-Mart had available and Columbia TN. was available. So I applied for that store, it was such a long shot I didn't even tell Ramona that I had applied for it at the time. A couple of weeks went by, 37 store managers had applied for the Columbia store. They told me I was in the top 5, then I told Ramona that I had applied. Obviously I got the store, we moved to Columbia a couple weeks before we had to move out of our Virginia house.

We had went down to Columbia, 2 weeks before we were to move down here, to find a house to rent. We looked all weekend, no luck. Everything was too small or rented out. Ramona had called a lady about a 4 bedroom house, she didn't answer. So we ran out of time and very discouraged we headed out of town not knowing where we would live when we got to Columbia in 2 weeks. Then Ramona's purse started talking. "Hello" "Hello". Without the phone ringing the last person Ramona had called was on the phone. She had a house in the country to rent and wanted us to come over and see it. We rented the house and moved to Columbia.

When I agreed to take the Columbia store I took a pay cut of about 15% because we were living close to Washington DC and they pay you a premium when you live next to a big city.

It was worth that pay cut to get closer to home. Ramona's parents are not in great shape and we wanted to be close to them.

When we finished 1998 and the stores profits were figured out (Which I receive a small percentage as a bonus) the Columbia store created a bonus for me of exactly the same amount above the old store as I had lost by coming to Columbia.

I am 100% convinced that God blessed us for being faithful and tithing like we are commanded to do.

I would like to leave you with just a thought. As parents, God trusts us to raise our children to fear him and to serve in his kingdom. I think this is the most important thing any of us will ever do. Our job is getting tougher everyday, the devil is on the throne in this world and it becomes more evil everyday. Paul warned of this in 2nd Timothy Chapter 3 verses 1-4. Paul also wrote the answer for us. What we need to do as parents to train our children 2nd Timothy Chapter 3 versus 14-17. What Paul is saying is to teach our children God's word.

As a person who grew up without God I can tell you that I missed out on a lot. I would encourage every parent to bring your children to church every time the doors are open. By doing this we can arm our children with God's protective armor. If we don't we leave them alone in this wicked world to fend for themselves.

The story you just read was what I spoke to my church members about. Again I thought I should share my story with my family. What I want you to know is that God loves you and he wants you to go to heaven, (I have enclosed a copy of scripture, Luke 16 verses 19-31).

LUKE

CHAPTER 16

1 And he said also unto his disciples, There was a certain rich man, which had a steward; and the same was accused unto him that he had wasted his goods.

2 And he called him, and said unto him, How is it that I hear this of thee? give an account of thy stewardship; for thou mayest be no longer steward.

3 Then the steward said within himself, What shall I do? for my lord taketh away from me the stewardship: I cannot dig; to beg I am ashamed.

4 I am resolved what to do, that, when I am put out of the stewardship, they may receive me into their houses.

5 So he called every one of his lord's debtors *unto him,* and said unto the first, How much owest thou unto my lord?

6 And he said, An hundred measures of oil. And he said unto him, Take thy bill, and sit down quickly, and write fifty.

7 Then said he to another, And how much owest thou? And he said, An hundred measures of wheat. And he said unto him, Take thy bill, and write fourscore.

8 And the lord commended the unjust steward, because he had done wisely: for the children of this world are in their generation wiser than the children of light.

9 And I say unto you, Make to yourselves friends of the mammon of unrighteousness; that, when ye fail, they may receive you into everlasting habitations.

10 He that is faithful in that which is least is faithful also in much: and he that is unjust in the least is unjust also in much.

11 If therefore ye have not been faithful in the unrighteous mammon, who will commit to your trust the true *riches*?

12 And if ye have not been faithful in that which is another man's, who shall give you that which is your own?

13 No servant can serve two masters: for either he will hate the one, and love the other; or else he will hold to the one, and despise the other. Ye cannot serve God and mammon.

14 And the Pharisees also, who were covetous, heard all these things: and they derided him.

15 And he said unto them, Ye are they which justify yourselves before men; but God knoweth your hearts: for that which is highly esteemed among men is abomination in the sight of God.

16 The law and the prophets *were* until John: since that time the kingdom of God is preached, and every man presseth into it.

17 And it is easier for heaven and earth to pass, than one tittle of the law to fail.

18 Whosoever putteth away his wife, and marrieth another, committeth adultery: and whosoever marrieth her that is put away from *her* husband committeth adultery.

19 There was a certain rich man, which was clothed in purple and fine linen, and fared sumptuously every day:

20 And there was a certain beggar named Lazarus, which was laid at his gate, full of sores,

21 And desiring to be fed with the crumbs which fell from the rich man's table: moreover the dogs came and licked his sores.

22 And it came to pass, that the beggar died, and was carried by the angels into Abraham's bosom: the rich man also died, and was buried;

23 And in hell he lift up his eyes, being in torments, and seeth Abraham afar off, and Lazarus in his bosom.

24 And he cried and said, Father Abraham, have mercy on me, and send Lazarus, that he may dip the tip of his finger in water, and cool my tongue; for I am tormented in this flame.

25 But Abraham said, Son, remember that thou in thy lifetime receivedst thy good things, and likewise Lazarus evil things: but now he is comforted, and thou art tormented.

26 And beside all this, between us and you there is a great gulf fixed: so that they which would pass from hence to you cannot; neither can they pass to us, that *would come* from thence.

27 Then he said, I pray thee therefore, father, that thou wouldest send him to my father's house:

28 For I have five brethren; that he may testify unto them, lest they also come into this place of torment.

29 Abraham saith unto him, They have Moses and the prophets; let them hear them.

30 And he said, Nay, father Abraham: but if one went unto them from the dead, they will repent.

31 And he said unto him, If they hear not Moses and the prophets, neither will they be persuaded, though one rose from the dead.

This story tells of a man who is in hell and wants to warn his family how terrible it is down there. I want to do the same thing. Thru out the Bible God tells us how awful hell is and that we are all going to hell unless we accept Jesus Christ at our personal savior.

I know that I will go to heaven and I know that it would be awful to think of any member of my family going to hell. So I ask you, if you die tonight do you know where you will spend eternity? If you don't know the answer to this question I will tell you it, you will go to hell and be tormented forever.

Jesus died for each of us. He was born to a virgin, walked and preached on earth 33 years, was crucified for our sins and died on the cross, then he was resurrected and is now on the throne in heaven. It is simple if you want to go to heaven all you have to do is to pray to Jesus Christ.

(1) Admit you are a sinner and ask God to forgive you.
(2) Acknowledge that he was born to a virgin, was crucified and died on a cross for your sins, and arose out the grave after 3 days and is in heaven on the throne now.
(3) Ask Jesus to forgive you and to come into your life.

It is that simple and my prayer is that every member of my family will accept Jesus and will go to heaven.

If I can be any help to you call me 931-381-6578 or write:

828 Rand Way
Columbia, TN 38401

May God Bless You!!!!

Richard Baud
3-1-2000

P.S. If you are not comfortable talking to me. Go to any Baptist Church and tell the preacher you want to be saved and God will take it from there.

I mentioned in an earlier chapter that my only daughter Katie had went down the aisle at age 7. At that time, we all thought she had been saved but at a revival service in November 1999, Katie realized that she was not saved and on 11-2-99 she asked Jesus to save her, and he did. She was baptized on 11-7-1999. This still left my son Richard, Jr. who was not saved. This was my passion, my top priority. I could not rest until he had been saved. My son had been going thru a lot of problems, During this time like all other times, I encouraged my son to look to the Lord for answers. I told him the only person he could always count on and never be disappointed in was our Lord Jesus Christ, he will never fail. He is there for you and me when those around fail or betray you.

Well, Richard Jr. finally started going to a local church in Robinson and started talking things over with the local preacher. Then on Sunday 9-16-2001 Richard, Jr. called me. He said "Dad I went to church this morning and the preacher was saying things that went right thru me. His words touched something inside me, and I felt the Lord telling me it was time. I never felt like this before. I started crying loudly and my friend Rod went with me down the aisle. I spoke to the preacher, knelt down and ask Jesus to forgive me and save me, and dad he did. I was saved today!!!"

As I listened to my son, I knew that God had answered all of my prayers for my son. I knew that my children would all go to heaven when they die, words cannot express what a relief that is. All I can say is THANK YOU LORD, PRAISE GOD, THANK YOU LORD.

It is amazing to me that my family's salvation began by an innocent question from an eight-year-old boy "Daddy what does that T stand for"

The circle closed for my immediate family on 9-16-2001, when the last member of my immediate family accepted the Lord. But as a Christian I am commanded to spread the Gospel and witness to others about the Lord Jesus Christ.

Life seems to take unexpected turns all the time. I realize more all the time that many of these twists and turns are part of God's plan to strengthen us and make use of his children.

In October of 2000 I received a call from my older brother,sounds normal but I hadn't heard from him in ten years. I really didn't know if I would ever hear from him again and frankly, I didn't care if I did or didn't. You see he, just like our oldest brother Danny had been in trouble half their lives, in and out of jail/prison. This particular brother had stolen from everyone including his family and me in particular. So when I got this call I was surprised and apprehensive.

He said "I'm out of prison and in a half-way house in Birmingham, Alabama. I've accepted the Lord and want to turn my life around." We talked for a while off and on for the next few months. My trust and faith in him was and still is zero. I believe nothing he says and only part of what I see, for he was the biggest liar I ever knew. But, thru prayer I sought Gods' will and I was lead to help him turn his life around. he had obviously had a life changing conversion because in the past he was so bad and my older brother clearly had come a long way. God put him in a great place. He was working for the church at Brook Hills. The pastor and others helped my older brother learn about how to behave and live his life in an acceptable manner. As I said earlier I was lead by the Lord to help my older brother and everything that I have done or will do is out of Christian love and a sense of duty as a child of God.

Events to come in the next few months helped me know how important it is to do whatever I can to reach out to others while I can before it is too late.

On the evening of March 13, 2001, I was working my normal late shift at Walmart when my wife Ramona, called me and said, "I have some bad news for you, your oldest brother Danny is dead." I don't remember much about the rest of that week. I was in a daze, my whole life changed. Danny was my first sibling to die, and it was a shock to believe he could be dead at 45. Danny had a rough life, like my older brother he was in trouble with the law a lot. Danny had been out of jail for a couple of years. Mainly because he had a crippling accident a couple of years ago, which left him barely able to get around. Danny was a drifter. He lived in his van and traveled back and forth "from where my mother and siblings lived", to Alabama and Florida where it was warmer, and he liked to go. Danny seemed like he was satisfied with his life. Danny used to stop by Columbia, Tn. and see me on the way back to Illinois. Mainly I guess to "borrow" money for gas or food. The last time I seen Danny was on Wednesday 3-7-2001. He went back to layaway "at Walmart" and had them call me there. I met Danny and talked for a few minutes (as always I was very busy and pressed for time.) So I asked Danny where he was going, he said he was heading south and might try to see my older brother (Danny's younger brother), because he knew he was out of prison. Danny as always needed something "do you guys carry a propane heater because I use propane to heat my van and my current heater smells like _____?" We looked for a heater but couldn't find one, so he said, "can you buy me a couple of propane tanks?" I gave him a $20 bill and said goodbye, I never knew this was the last time I would see him alive.

A couple of years prior to this, when Danny came to see me, I took him to my house to meet my wife and children and gave him a cup of coffee. He sat in my living room and said he liked the way he lived and wouldn't change it if he could, he loved traveling with his dog. I asked Danny if he died today where would you spend eternity? He said, "Rick we were all saved when we were young the few times we went to church." I do not know if my brother went to heaven, God knows I hope he did, but I know when I was a child, I was not saved regardless of any words I might have said back then. My prayer is that either Danny really was saved back then or was saved when he was crippled or the many times, he talked to preachers that helped him over the years.

The only thing that I know, is that I could have done more to witness to my oldest brother. I know that only God can save you thru Jesus Christ, but we are commanded to do our part. I still have even today a copy of the letter I sent to my extended family on 3-1-2000, addressed to Danny Ruffner, this was never given to him. I will keep this as long as I live to remind me that we only have a limited time to do our part to witness to our love ones, once they are dead time is up.

This brings me back to my older brother, since Danny died, my older brother has moved to Tennessee where he is closer to me and closer to his other family in Illinois. Most of my family thinks I am absurd for helping my older brother, but I know what they don't, even though he is very troubled and is not even close to being where he should be or needs to be, I believe in miracles,and I know all things are possible with God. I will continue to do what I can do to help him . My most important part is to pray for him and to ask God to help him to continue to improve his life and show him the correct path. I realize that even though he may be saved, he still has his old body and his past experiences, and the devil will battle him every inch of the way. So to my older brother, I can encourage you that even though man may give up on you God will never forsake you.

In an earlier chapter I told you that I would tell you more about our current church in Columbia, Tn., Northside Baptist Church. I've heard a lot in the years since I have been saved about how many churches are cold and lifeless, so I thank God for sending our family to Columbia, Tn. and making our church home Northside Baptist Church. When we came to Columbia in May of 1998, we tried all the local Baptist churches most of them a couple of times. There was something different about Northside Baptist Church. When we first walked into the sanctuary, we were greeted by almost everyone in the room, there is a warm, friendly atmosphere in the church. The church members truly welcome you and are glad you are there, and when the pastor John Rushing started to preach, we knew we were at a God-fearing Bible believing church. The pastor is a man of God, who tells it like it is regardless if it is popular or politically correct. The church members of our church were very blessed to have this man as our pastor. As the pastor would say our purpose as a church is to spread the gospel and help others find our Lord Jesus Christ as their savior.

For many years I have been conflicted over the amount of time I spend at my job as a store manager of a Walmart store, but I have felt that somehow it is part of God's plan for my life. Many times our pastor preached that you should use your vocation as a mission field to help others learn about Jesus Christ and lead them to salvation. As store manager I was limited to what I could say or do but I have been able to express my opinion and share some of my personal experiences thru a monthly newsletter our store had, which we used to communicate to all of our store associates. I have included a couple of examples of those newsletters.

The Wal-Mart Smiley Town News
December 1999
Volume 1 Issue 6

A Note From Richard,

Dear Wal-Mart Associates,

While Christmas is drawing near, we at Wal-Mart are busy unloading trucks, stocking shelves, ringing up customers and helping shoppers in the store. I would like to take a moment to reflect upon the true meaning of Christmas, and to share an experience that happened to me at a Wal-Mart that changed my life.

The reason for the season is Jesus Christ. Almost 2000 years ago Jesus Christ was born, sent by God to be a Savior to all mankind. I think on his birthday that it is only right to remember the great sacrifice of his death by crucifixion, and the following resurrection. He did this all for our sakes, so that anyone who calls on his name can be saved and have eternal everlasting life. In relation to this, I will tell you of a personal experience, and since Wal-Mart has been a very important part of my life for a long time, it is only fitting that it occurred at Wal-Mart.

It was a busy Friday in the middle of December 1996. While I was the Store Manager of the Wal-Mart in Manassa, Virginia, one of our Department Managers, Lennette Hurt, gave me a poem entitled, "Twas The Night Before Jesus Came." As I read this poem I was crushed. For the first time in my life I realized that I would never see Jesus or go to Heaven because I was not saved.

The next two days Jesus worked on me. I felt his presence and I was convicted and I knew that I needed to be saved. That Sunday, December 15, 1996, as our preacher gave the invitation, I walked to the front of the church and asked Jesus to forgive me for my sins, and I gave my life to Jesus! That same day I was baptized, and am proud to say that my children have all been saved and now I look forward to the day Jesus will return.

May God Bless You All,
Richard Baud
12/15/99

Richard's poem. It is located on the second page of this newsletter.

TWAS THE NIGHT BEFORE
JESUS CAME

Twas the night before Jesus came and all through the house,
Not a creature was praying, not one in the house.
Their Bibles were lain on the shelf without care,
In hopes that Jesus would not come there.

The children were dressing to crawl into bed,
Not once ever kneeling or bowing a head.
And Mom in the rocker with Baby on her lap,
Was watching the Late Show while I took a nap.

When out of the East there arose such a clatter,
I sprang to my feet to see what was the matter.
Away to the window I flew like a flash!
Tore open the shutters and threw up the sash!

When what to my wondering eyes should appear,
But angels proclaiming that Jesus was here!
With a light like the sun sending forth a bright ray,
I knew in a moment this must be the day.

The light of his face made me cover my heard,
It was Jesus returning just like he said.
And though I possessed worldly wisdom and wealth,
I cried when I saw him in spite of myself.

In The Book of Life which he held in his hand,
Was written the name of every saved man.
He spoke not a word as he searched for my name,
When he said "It's not here." My head hung in shame.

The people whose names had been written with love,
He gathered to take to his Father above.
With those who were ready he arose without a sound,
While all the rest were left standing around.

I fell to my knees, but it was too late,
I had waited too long and thus sealed my fate.
I stood and I cried as they arose out of sight,
Oh, if only I had been ready tonight!

In the words of this poem the meaning is clear,
The coming of Jesus is drawing near.
There's only one life and when comes the last call,
We'll find that the Bible was true after all!

The Wal-Mart Smiley Town News
April - 2001
Volume 1 Issue 20

A Note From Richard:

Dear Wal-Mart Associates,

In this month's issue, I would like to take the opportunity for some personal reflection.

Over the past three years I have been impressed with how this store's Associates come together to support their fellow Associates. Through sickness, death, or other personal tragedy our Associates are there in times of need. Unfortunately, I now know this support first hand.

In March my oldest brother, Danny, died in his sleep at the age of forty-five. There had been no sign that he was ill, or was having any health problems. This personal tragedy was a shock to me and my entire family. I want to thank all of you who sent cards, letters, expressed sympathy, or let me know that you are praying for my family. Your thoughtfulness is very much appreciated.

From experience I would like to give you some advice of a personal nature. When someone you love dies it is too late to tell them you love them. Don't miss one chance to spend time with your family. Slow down, reflect on your life, and know what is important. Don't be petty or hold grudges. And don't try to win the argument. Life is short, so do yourself a favor and live today like it is your last day on earth.

Most importantly know where you are going to spend eternity! Since Easter is next Sunday I would be remiss if I did not give credit where credit is due. I want to tell you about a friend of mine. His name is Jesus who was sent from Heaven, by God, in the form of a baby born unto a Virgin. He walked the earth thirty-three years spreading the Gospel, telling the world of God's love. He was crucified on a cross and died for our sins.

That is only part of his story. After three days, Jesus rose again, defeating death. He lives today, offering us eternal life if we admit we are sinners and acknowledge that Jesus Christ is God's son who died and rose gain after three days. If you ask Jesus to save you, he promises to do just that.

Again I appreciate all that each and everyone of you do. Not only by doing your job but by being a family to your fellow Associates.

Thank you, and may God bless you.
Richard Baud
April 07, 20001

Business Page Alert!

The **Business Page** will return in the next issue. For now, all associates should be focused on completing the Grass Roots Survey. For assistance contact a member of management or the **Personnel Office**.

On 9-11-2001 a horrible event took place that shook the entire world, terrorists attacked America and killed thousands of innocent people. If you are to ever have a wake-up call, something that will let you know that you are mortal and will die someday, this is it!!! Recently I sent my extended family a letter once again pleading for them to get their lives straight and ask Jesus to save them before it is everlasting too late. I am enclosing a copy of the letter I sent dated 11-5-01, I have also enclosed a copy of the card with step by step instructions.

Dear Family Members:

Since the September 11th attack on the United States, I am compelled to write to you. Thousands of innocent people died in an instant. They were normal Americans doing their normal jobs, living like they were going to live a long time. Some were working on their computers, some were sweeping the floors, some were repairing telephones, and some were on break drinking coffee. Some people were just walking nearby. Of course the thing that they all had in common, was that they didn't know that they would die that day. We that still live today have an opportunity to get our lives in order and be ready when we die. I ask you now, do you know where you would go if you died today? If you do thank God for that!!!!! But if you don't please listen to what I am saying, God has a plan-He sent his only son Jesus Christ to die for me and you, so that you can be saved and have eternal everlasting life. All that you had to do is believe that Jesus is the Son of God, believe that he was crucified on that cross, died, defeated hell and death, and rose again in three days. Believe this, ask Jesus to forgive you for your sins and ask Jesus to save you and He will. Once this is done you can have that internal peace, and you will know that when you die you will go to Heaven. I am also sending you a small card, one side shows God's Plan of Salvation, the other side shows you what to do once you have been saved. The Bible tells us that God wants everyone to be saved, but you have to make the decision, and remember we are not promised tomorrow.

Thank you for listening to me.

May God Bless You,

Richard Baud
11-5-2001

THE ROMAN ROAD

Jesus prepared for us a simple plan of salvation. Presented in the Book of Romans of the Holy Bible, this outline will show you step by step how to be saved.

ROMANS 3:23
"For all have sinned, and come short of the glory of God." -- ALL have sinned --

ROMANS 5:8
"But God commendeth his love toward us, in that, while we were yet sinners. Christ died for us." -- ALL are loved --

ROMANS 6:23
"For the wages of sin is death, but the gift of God is eternal life through Jesus Christ our Lord." -- The PAYMENT for sin is death, separation from God forever. But salvation is a GIFT from God, not earned by going to church, baptism, good works, etc. --

ROMANS 10:9, 10
"That if thou shalt confess with thy mouth the Lord Jesus, and shalt believe in thine heart that God hath raised him from the dead, THOU SHALT BE SAVED." "For with the heart man believeth unto righteousness; and with the mouth confession is made unto salvation." -- Just BELIEVE and RECEIVE --

ROMANS 10:13
"For WHOSOEVER shall call upon the name of the Lord SHALL BE SAVED."

AFTER FOLLOWING THE PLAN OF SALVATION LEAD THEM IN THIS PRAYER

Dear Lord Jesus, I'm a Sinner -- I'm Lost. I Need to be Saved. I Want to be Saved. If You Will Save Me, I'll Give You My Life. Thank You Jesus for Saving Me.

–– After praying this prayer, go over the scriptures on
the other side of this card ––

THE NEXT STEPS

Now that you have accepted Christ as your own personal Saviour, what
next?

1. ASSURANCE (1 John 5:13)

"These things have I written unto you that believe on the name of the
Son of God: that YE MAY KNOW that ye have eternal life, and that
ye may believe on the name of the Son of God."

2. CONFESS (Matthew 10:32, 33)

"Whosoever therefore shall confess me before men, him will I confess
also before my Father which is in heaven." "But whosoever shall deny
me before men, him will I also deny before my Father which is in
heaven."

3. BAPTISM (Acts 2:38, 41)

"Repent, and be baptized every one of you." "Then they that gladly
received his word were baptized."

4. WITNESS (Psalms 107:2)

"Let the redeemed of the Lord say so." - Tell others about Christ -

5. GIVE WEEKLY (1 Corinthians 16:2)

"Upon the first day of the week let every one of you lay by him in store,
as God hath prospered him, that there be no gathering when I come."

6. DEVOTION (II Timothy 2:15)

"Study to show thyself approved unto God, a workman that needeth
not to be ashamed, rightly dividing the word of truth."
- Read your Bible, pray and share your faith every day -

My Walmart career would start on Dec. 30, 1980, and end 11-19-2020. I would work hard and many hours to be able to succeed at my job, but it was not until I was saved on Dec. 15, 1996 that I realized that I was not really in charge and my success in life would be guided by my belief in God, and my attempt to live in a way that would be pleasing to God. In an upcoming chapter titled "Walmart" I will explain in more detail of my journey thru Walmart. For now I will end this chapter by saying that God has been so good to me.

CHAPTER 4

FAT

This chapter will be focused on me being fat and my battle to overcome my history of bad eating habits and an effort to return to a more normal weight.

I grew up in a large family that was very poor, so as a child overeating was not a problem. There was not enough food around to overeat. So, I was normal weight to a bit skinny all the way thru high school. Once I graduated high school and left home, I immediately developed poor eating habits and started adding pounds. My jobs were in retail and included working evenings, so my problem continued to get worse as I overate my way to getting fat. As time went on, I would try different diets, they did not help. I would lose a few pounds, then gain the pounds back plus a few.

As my weight problems grew worse, I learned to live with being called names like rotund, chubby, big man, also I got used to shopping at big and tall shops, I would always say that I was tall.

My weight got so bad that taking flights to business meetings meant me wondering if the seat belt would be big enough to fit around me or if I would have to ask the flight attendant to give me a seat belt extension (this was always embarrassing to me.)

At the end of this chapter, I've included my story of how I was able to finally figure out how to overcome my weight problem in 2006 and 2007. I was able to lose 130 pounds in nine months by developing my own diet and exercise plan and sticking to it. The key to my weight loss back in 2006 and 2007 was to have the proper motivation to start a plan and to stick to it, you can read about this at the end of this chapter.

Unfortunately, after I lost 130 pounds in nine months in 2006 and

2007, I did not keep my weight off. I started off good, maintaining my weight thru 2008 and then I started to relax and exercised less and ate and snacked more. So gradually I picked up the pounds as life continued to happen. My job got tougher (more about that in the next chapter). My mother died in 2011 and all of our children left home, one at a time to start their own lives. All these factors led me back to being the fat man again. At the peak of my weight before the 2006/2007 diet and exercise plan, I weighed 363 pounds. By Feb. 1, 2020, I was back up to 355 pounds. As I have previously stated you must have the proper motivation to succeed on any diet and exercise plan. On Feb. 1, 2020, I began to eat less and snack less and started to get back to better habits. Honestly, I was not greatly motivated at that time, and I made only small efforts towards losing weight. This continued until Nov. 19, 2020, when I left the employment of Walmart where I had worked for 37 years. Once I was not employed, I could focus on me, and my diet became a lot better. I cut out most snacks and controlled what I ate and when I ate my food. I gradually was able to lose 50 pounds between Feb. 1, 2020 and July 1, 2021.

For years I would listen to the radio to a chiropractor who was talking about whole health and how his chiropractic offices would focus on your entire health, including chiropractic care and nutrition. I was very curious about this practice but frankly I was scared of chiropractors.

One day I got brave and called the doctor that I had listened to for years and scheduled an appointment at one of his offices. This turned out to be a very good thing. At this office I was shown x-rays of how my lower back and my neck were showing deterioration, they explained what was happening and where I was headed if I did not reverse my current course. They also came up with a plan to fix my neck and lower back.

I am a skeptical person by nature, so I took what they were telling me with a grain of salt, but I was convinced enough to overcome my fear of chiropractors and give it a try.

I have been on a plan with this office since July 1, 2021. Gradually my neck and back are improving. I am still scared every time the chiropractor does any corrections on my neck and back, but I call on God to protect me, so far, he has.

After I had been with my chiropractor and their office for a week, I had a consultation with their health advisor and was shown their plan for getting healthy by eating correctly. This includes eating healthy food and taking some quality supplements. I have included in this chapter a copy of their entire plan. Exactly what they gave me on July 7, 2021. So, I decided to jump in and try their diet plan. I like things very simple, so I took their basic ideas and choices, and I made my own diet. This is a simple plan and something I can stick with. The following is what I eat daily.

Breakfast: One orange, one banana, and blueberries /raspberries. All organic.

Lunch: One cucumber, one red tomato, one apple. All organic. Also I have four ounces of natural turkey breast.

Supper: Two pieces of baked salmon (wild caught). A frozen bag of Birdseye vegetables. To mix it up I rotate between the fish and free-range chicken thighs and fried eggs and toast.

Also daily I drink 100 ounces of water, including two glasses of water with lemon squeezed into the water. The water helps keep the body flushed of all toxins, etc. In addition to what I eat and drink I take these supplements daily. These are attached.

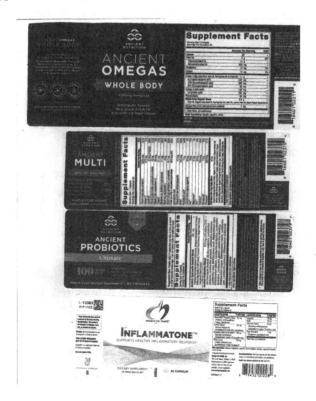

So I started this new plan on July 9, 2021. I only eat what was in my plan for breakfast, lunch, and super, with an occasional splurge when eating with my kids and grandchildren. This is a big key, you have to be able to get right back on the plan the next day or this or any plan will not work. I only drink water, I have eliminated all sodas and other types of drink from my diet.

I also begin to walk every morning, I started slow but now I am walking three to four miles each day, including going down and back up a very steep hill at our apartment complex. So, between my walking and my new diet plan I had lost 28 pounds by Aug 7, 2021. Remember I started on July 9, 2021, as I complete my book my current weight is 249 pounds. So, I have lost 106 pounds since I begin my diet on Feb. 1, 2020.

So here I am on a new plan that appears to be working. The same thing that is making this diet and exercise plan work is what made my diet and exercise plan in 2006/2007 work. It takes dedication and motivation. As you read my story from 2006/2007 you will see what motivated me then. As for my current diet and exercise plan, here is what motivates me now. First, I want to be able to spend good quality time with my children and grandchildren. Second, I want to be able to be healthy enough to help out in my community using my hard-earned experience to help others. Third, I want to be able to be used by God to help spread his word and see people saved.

To anyone reading this, that wishes to do anything meaningful in life, you have to have the proper dedication and motivation. This can be many things among them, (1) to get healthy, (2) to live longer, (3) to set a good example for (a) for kids (b) your grandkids (c) others you are close to.

As I promised earlier in this chapter, I'm adding the plan that I was given from Mission Health (chiropractor). I used this plan to develop a plan that works for me.

EAT BY DESIGN 101

What is eating by design about?

Eating by design is eating the way God created our bodies to be fueled. By following a whole food-based diet and leading physically active lives, our ancestors presumably had much lower rates of lifestyle diseases, such as obesity, diabetes and heart disease.

The diet varied depending on what was available and where in the world people lived. Some ate low carb high fat diets while others followed diets rich in lots of plant foods.

Consider this as a general guideline. Listen to your body and pay attention to how your body communicates with you.

Here are the basics:

Eat:	Avoid:
grass-fed meats	all processed foods
free range poultry	sugar
eggs	soft drinks
raw cheese (goat & sheep are especially good)	grains
grass-fed butter/ghee	most dairy products
vegetables	legumes
fruits	artificial sweeteners
nuts	vegetable oils
seeds	margarine
herbs & spices	trans fats
healthy fats	
clean oils	

Foods to avoid:

Sugar and high-fructose corn syrup: soft drinks, fruit juices, table sugar, candy, pastries, ice cream etc

Grains: breads, pastas, wheat, spelt, rye, barely, rice etc

Legumes: beans, lentils, peas, coffee etc

Dairy: especially low fat processed dairy (milk, sour cream, cheese)

Vegetable oil: soybean, canola, sunflower, cottonseed, corn, safflower

Trans fats: margarine, chips, fried foods, hydrogenated or partially hydrogenated oils

Artificial sweeteners: aspartame, sucralose, cyclamates, saccharin, acesulfame potassium

Highly processed foods: everything labeled as "diet" or "low fat" or anything that has additives, MSG (monosodium glutamate)

A simple guideline, if it comes in a box or package and looks like it was made in a factory- do not eat it.

Start reading labels and avoid anything that contains ingredients listed above.

Foods to eat:

Meat: grass-fed beef, lamb, venison, bison, chicken, turkey, organic pork

Fish and seafood: wild caught alaskan salmon, trout, haddock, shrimp, shellfish, etc

Eggs: choose free range/pastured eggs, farm fresh is always best

Vegetables: broccoli, cabbage, brussel sprouts, kale, lettuce, swiss chard, bok choy, green onions, cilantro, parsley, cauliflower, carrots, sweet potatoes, squash, zucchini, cucumbers, tomatoes, peppers, eggplant, onions etc

Fruits: blueberries, blackberries, strawberries, raspberries, golden berries, gogi berries, apples, pears, bananas, oranges, lemon, limes, grapefruit *organic when possible

Nuts & Seeds: almonds, cashews, macadamia, Brazil, chia, hemp, flax, coconut etc

Healthy fats & oils: extra virgin olive oil, virgin coconut oil, grass-fed butter/ghee, avocado oil etc

Salt & spices: pink himalayan salt, black pepper, all organic herbs and spices

Vinegars: apple cider vinegar, balsamic vinegar, red wine vinegar

Sweeteners: dates, maple syrup, raw honey, coconut sugar, organic stevia extract (not powder), monk fruit

Wine: high quality dry organic wine, red, white or rose

Dark chocolate: organic dairy free dark chocolate at least 70%

Resources
**www.draxe.com www.getbetterwellness.
com www.nomnompaleo.com** ave

SAMPLE MEAL PLAN

Breakfast

egg & veggie scramble with bacon
- 2 pastured eggs
- 1/2 cup mushrooms
- 1/2 cup chopped red bell peppers
- 1/4 cup chopped red onion
- 1 cup spinach
- 1 tbsp butter/ghee
- 1 tsp salt
- Organic bacon

Saute mushrooms, peppers, onions and spinach in a skillet for 10-15 minutes on medium heat.
Turn heat to low and add whisked eggs.
Sprinkle with salt.

Bake bacon at 425 for 20 minutes or until desired.

Lunch

garden salad with left over grilled chicken
- 4 cups spring mix
- 1/2 cup chopped cucumber
- 1/2 cup chopped cherry tomatoes
- 1/2 cup shredded carrots
- 4-6 oz. left over grilled chicken
- Drizzle with extra virgin olive oil, red wine vinegar, salt and pepper

Mix all ingredients in large bowl.

Snack

Dates & Nut Butter
- 3-4 pitted dates
- 2 tbsp. Nut butter (sunbather, almond butter and cashew butter)
- Sprinkle of salt

Dinner

Baked Salmon & Sautéed Veggies
- 1 wild caught salmon fillet
- 1-2 tbsp grass-fed butter
- 1 tsp dill
- 1 tsp parsley
- 1 tsp garlic powder
- 1 tsp salt
- 1 tsp black pepper

Sautéed Veggies
- 1/2 cup mushrooms
- 1/2 cup sliced bell peppers
- 1/2 cup chopped broccoli
- 1 tbsp ghee/coconut oil
- 1 tsp salt
- 1 tsp black pepper

Pre-heat oven to 350. Rub butter, herbs, salt and pepper on salmon fillet. Bake for 15-17 minutes.
Saute veggies until desired (15-20 minutes).

SUPPLEMENT PLAN

Probiotic (100 bill CFUs)	2 Capsules	Take At Night
Multi Vitamin	1 Capsules	Take In The Morning
Inflammatone	2 Capsules	Take During The Day
Omega	3 Capsules	Take At Night

Further Recommendations

Drink 20oz fresh bone broth everyday.

Drink 90-120oz water each day. Add
freshly squeezed lemon juice to
promote liver health and help balance your body's pH levels.

Start cooking with virgin coconut oil
or ghee (clarified butter).

Switch your salt- make sure your salt is
unprocessed. Pink Himalayan salt
is the best option.

bone broth brand - bonafied (freezer @ whole foods)

I also promised that I would have a copy of my story of weight loss from 2006/2007. This story starts on the next page.

You should note that the plan from 2006/2007 is totally different from the 2021 plan, but both rely on serious dedication to the plan and are motivated by people I love and want to show my example of how to overcome any obstacle.

I DID IT AND YOU CAN TOO!!!!

Before	After

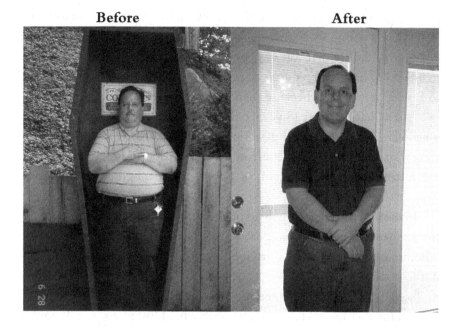

On July 4th, 2006 I declared my independence from being overweight. Since then I have lost over 130 pounds. That is over 130 pounds in 9 months!!!

Over the last several weeks I have had so many people ask me the same question "How have you lost so much weight and in such a small amount of time?"

My job puts me in the public everyday and I believe that I can be an example for other overweight people to follow, so I am compelled to tell my story.

I did it and you can too!!!

MY STORY

I will begin by telling you a little about how I arrived at being overweight. When I was young I was always a normal size to a little bit skinny. I was born into a family that was very poor and most of the time my mother struggled to have enough to feed me and my seven brothers and sisters; so I could not overeat because there was never anything left to overeat.

After I left home at 18 years old, I started to overeat. I basically ate whatever I wanted to and I developed bad habits that would lead me to weight gain. I worked in retail and had to work odd hours which had me getting off work at 10 p.m. or 11 p.m. and eating before I went to sleep at night.

I continued these bad habits for the next 27 years, gradually going from normal weight to being extremely overweight. Like most people who are overweight, I have tried every type of diet and exercise plan in the book.

Some of these plans helped me lose a little weight but once I grew tired of the diet I would always gain back what I lost plus some. I would wait a while then try again. I would convince myself that I needed to lose weight for various reasons: health, energy level, or just to be able to shop for clothes at a normal clothing store. Even though I tried hard to make it happen I just could not do it. It seemed like nothing would ever change. I was destined to continue to be overweight forever.

For the last five years or so, I didn't even try to lose weight. I had given up on diet programs. I was content to just maintain my weight. I figured that after I have my 1st heart attack I would get serious about it and then lose weight. This all changed one day, our family had just returned from our vacation in Gatlinburg, TN. And two things happened that would finally give me the answer to my weight problem.

First I heard my son talk about gaining over 30 pounds in a short time, then my daughter complained that no matter how hard she tried, she could not get to the size she wanted to get to.

Now let me tell you I felt terrible. I knew that I was responsible for my children heading towards a life of being overweight. I had been able to rationalize my being overweight but I knew that I could not just stand by and watch my children go thru the same thing that I had dealt with most of my life.

When something happens to you its one thing but watching it happen to your children is another thing indeed. I made the decision immediately; I will either lose weight and show my children how to lose weight and how to keep it off, or I will die trying.

At the time I didn't know how much weight I could lose, but I knew that I must do it and do it now. I figured that if I could show them the way and set the example for them, that they would follow me and have a better life.

MY STORY

At the end of my story of how I have been able to lose so much weight in such a small amount of time, I have added information on the amount of calories various foods have.

Well, I decided to do it the old fashion way. First I decided to limit the amount of calories I consumed everyday and start exercising. I am the type of person who has to plan things out and follow a plan. So I came up with a daily plan as to exactly what to eat at each meal, and a daily plan as to what type of exercise and how long to exercise each day.

I made up my plans and executed them like never before. This time I had a new motivation. I was not losing weight for me; I was losing weight for my children.

Here is how my weight came off; on 7-4-2006 my starting weight was 363 pounds.

	8-28-06 – 324	11-11-06 – 287	1-24-07 – 255
7-12-06 – 360	8-30-06 – 320	11-15-06 – 286	2-17-07 – 254
7-14-06 – 356	9-3-06 – 319	11-22-06 – 285	2-18-07 – 252
7-15-06 – 353	9-6-06 – 315	11-26-06 – 283	2-21-07 – 250
7-17-06 – 352	9-8-06 – 314	11-29-06 – 281	2-27-07 – 249
7-18-06 – 347	9-11-06 – 313	12-5-06 – 280	2-28-07 – 248
7-19-06 – 346	9-13-06 – 311	12-13-06 – 278	3-2-07 – 247
7-21-06 – 343	9-16-06 – 309	12-20-06 – 276	3-6-07 – 245
8-2-06 – 338	9-27-06 – 306	12-21-06 – 275	3-14-07 – 243
8-9-06 – 333	10-3-06 – 302	12-24-06 – 274	3-18-07 – 242
8-12-06 – 331	10-15-06 – 299	12-25-06 – 272	3-21-07 – 240
8-17-06 – 330	10-18-06 – 298	12-27-06 – 269	4-4-07 – 239
8-19-06 – 329	10-22-06 – 297	1-2-07 – 267	4-9-07 – 238
8-12-06 – 327	10-23-06 – 295	1-3-07 – 264	4-10-07 – 237
8-17-06 – 330	10-25-06 – 294	1-4-07 – 263	4-11-07 – 236
8-19-06 – 329	10-29-06 – 293	1-17-07 – 262	4-18-07 – 233
8-23-06 – 327	10-30-06 – 292	1-19-07 – 261	
8-24-06 – 326	11-2-06 – 290	1-21 -07 – 260	
8-27-06 – 325	11-8-06 – 288	1-23-07 – 258	

I now have lost over 130 pounds and I feel the calling to help others do what I have done.

After lots of consideration I have embarked on a plan to help educate and motivate people.

MOTIVATION

I have now told you about my story and where I am coming from, now let me focus on you.

If you are serious about losing weight you will need to do a couple of things.

No. 1 Review how you got overweight in the first place.

No. 2 Decide if you are ready to make the total commitment to changing habits and losing weight.

No. 3 You will need motivation to get you started and to keep you going because this will be tough and it is not for the faint of heart. Like I told you earlier, I did not come to the point where I could finally get it done until I had something bigger than myself to push me to get started, and to keep me going thru the process of diet and exercise. So you need to do some soul searching and come up with your reason for losing weight. Is it your children, your spouse, your grandchildren, or something else? Whatever it is figure it out and get started on the next stage – the planning stage.

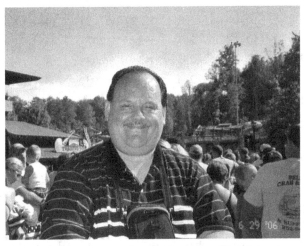

(BIG GUYS DAY AT THE PARK)

COMMITMENT

Let me tell you right now that if you do not have the proper motivation that is based on losing weight to set the example for others or to become healthy in order to be around to help support your children, or to play with your grandchildren, etc. If you do not have this amazing commitment then do not even bother getting started yet. Wait until you are totally committed and motivated to losing the weight and doing it now!!

ME AND MY DAUGHTER KATIE
BEFORE

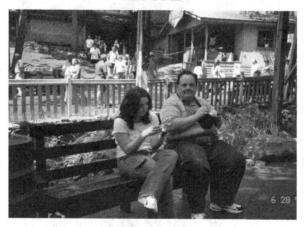

ME AND MY DAUGHTER KATIE
AFTER

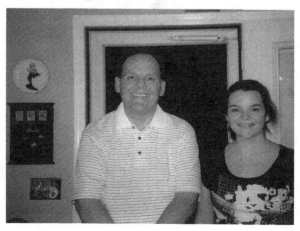

ME AND MY SON SAMUEL, BEFORE PICTURE

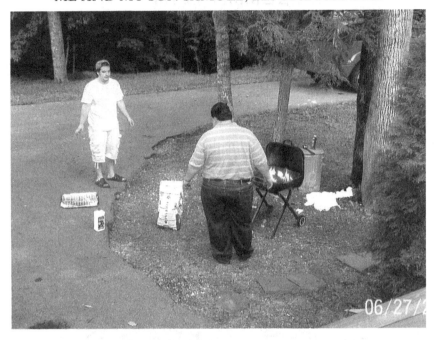

ME AND MY SON SAMUEL, AFTER PICTURE

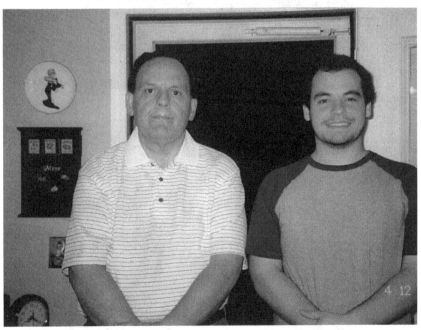

ME AND LAUREN, BEFORE PICTURE

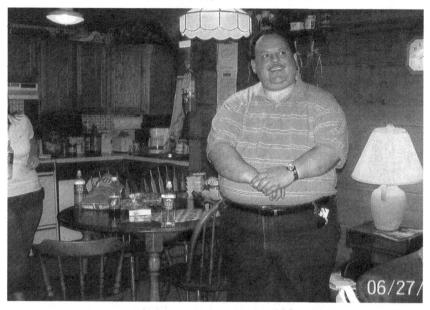

ME AND LAUREN, AFTER PICTURE

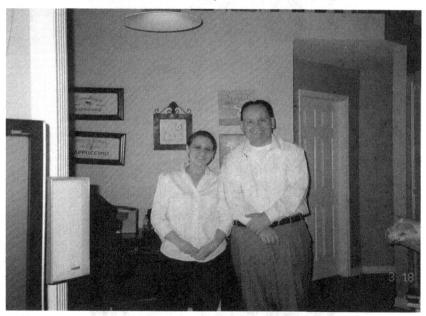

ME AND JOSH BEFORE

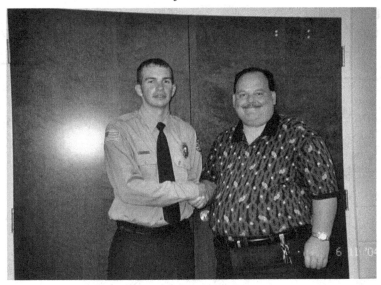

ME AND JOSH AFTER

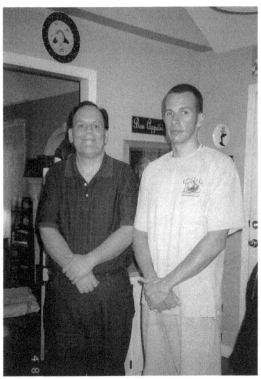

THE PLAN

Apparently you have made the commitment and are ready to get started on a plan. What I am going to do is to show you what I did and show you how to make your own plan. Before I show you my plan, let me tell you how I came up with it and why.

I knew before I started this diet and exercise plan that it must be different then my other diet plans and it must be something that I can get a quick start on, and something that I could stick with for the long term.

I decided to keep it simple. First I made a list of rules that I must follow:

1. I will eat and drink only what is on my daily meal plan.
2. I will follow my exercise plan exactly – no deviation.
3. I will eat nothing after 7 p.m.
4. I will eat no snacks like chips, candy bars, etc. I will stick to grapes, bananas, apples, and oranges when I must eat between meals.
5. In order not to get burnt out on my diet plan, once a month I will allow myself to have one day where I can eat out and not worry about counting calories.

The following is a copy of my daily diet plan for everyday of the week. A copy of my exercise plan for the days of the week. I had the time to exercise Saturday, Monday, Wednesday, and Thursday.

Daily Meal Plan

Saturday – Monday – Thursday
Breakfast: 2 Waffles with light butter and syrup
Coffee and water to drink

Lunch: Subway
Subway Club with American cheese and nothing else.
1 Bag of Lays Baked Chips
Drink – Water

Supper: 1 can of soup – no crackers
            Drink – Light Minute Maid

Snacks: 1 apple, 10-15 grapes

Sunday and Wednesday
Breakfast: None

Lunch: 1 can of soup – no crackers
            Drink – Water

Supper: 1 can of soup – no crackers
            Drink – Diet Lipton Tea

Snacks: 1 apple, 10-15 grapes

Tuesday and Friday
Breakfast: 1 sausage biscuit
            Drink – Coffee and water

Lunch: Subway
            Subway Club with American cheese and nothing else.
            1 small bag of Baked Lays chips
            Drink – Water

Supper: McDonalds – This is not healthy but I need to keep a
            variety in my diet.
            ValueMeal – normal size burger, French fries, Dr. Pepper

Snacks: Orange, banana

Daily Exercise Plan

Exercise on these days:

Saturday 7 p.m. – 2 hours mowing yard with push mower, if bad
weather go to treadmill – 3 miles.

Monday 7 p.m. – 3 miles on treadmill at 3 miles per hour speed.

Wednesday 10 a.m. – 2 hours mowing yard with push mower, if bad weather go to treadmill – 3 miles.

Thursday 7 p.m. – 3 miles on treadmill at 3 miles per hour speed.

Getting Your Plan Together

Before I start giving you advice, I need to proclaim that I am not a doctor, not a dietitian, not an expert on anything. What I am is a man who has struggled with being overweight for many years. I have finally figured out how to lose weight and I am willing to share how I did it with you.

I have debated on how to suggest that you come up with your plan, maybe these traditional ways:

1. Charts on height and weight
2. Recommendations from experts
3. Complicated formulas on protein vs. carbs

But instead I decided to keep it simple and go with what I did. After I decided to lose weight I started looking carefully at my habits.

1. What was I eating?
2. The times I was eating.
3. What I snacked on.
4. What I was drinking.

And my daughter who was 16 years old at the time said "Dad you need to pay attention to how many calories you are eating." After that tip from my daughter I started reading the information on cans and labels on packages on fast food, etc.

I soon discovered that this was a big key to losing weight. The amount of calories I was consuming daily was amazing. So I came up with a plan based on consuming less than 2000 calories a day. I already gave you my plan – so let's start with your plan.

I suggest that you come up with a plan based on limiting your calories to no more than 2000 a day. A simple way to figure your calorie needs is to multiply your current weight by 7, this will give you roughly your daily calorie needs.

Pick foods you like and that are readily available and plan out each meal. Remember, as you lose weight, recalculate your calorie needs and reduce the calories you consume daily.

I am providing you with a daily meal plan form. Fill this out for every day of the week, break down the amount of calories you will consume daily and split it up between breakfast, lunch, supper, and snacks.

Make sure you plan out the portions you can eat based on how many calories that food has. You must also remember that what you drink may have calories in it. For example, Dr. Pepper – 20 ounces has almost 300 calories. You should stick to water, coffee, unsweet tea, etc. Once you have written out your meal plan on the daily meal plan forms, take that days form with you and refer to it throughout the day to keep you on track.

DAILY MEAL CARD

Day of Week =
1 Breakfast

Maximum Calories =
2 Lunch

Maximum Calories =
3 Supper

Maximum Calories =
4 Snacks Allowed
Drinks =
Fruits =

5 Cannot eat or drink
anything else, not on card

6 Cannot eat or drink
anything after 7pm

Maximum Calories Allowed
Per Day =

You will find that two things will happen:

1. Some meals will not work out and you will need to be flexible and revise your daily meal plan regularly, but stick to total calories under 2000 a day.
2. After a few weeks, your routines will change and you will not have to carry the daily meal plan cards with you; it will become habit.

Now start on your exercise plans. First get the days of the week and times of the day that you can devote to exercise figured out. Then plan the type of exercise you will do. Consider unique and different exercises. I started by using my push mower to mow my hilly yard in the summer heat. You might have something like that you can do, or maybe ride a bike, push your baby in a stroller, or just get on the treadmill or exercise bike. Try lots of different things until you find something right for you. Then utilize the daily exercise card to document your planned exercise.

No. 1 – Day of week
No. 2 – Time of exercise
No. 3 – Type of exercise
No. 4 – Amount of time you will exercise

I suggest that you start slow. If you decide to use the treadmill, maybe walk on it for one mile at a slow pace. Then gradually build up to 2 or 3 miles and increase your speed as you feel stronger. Remember to stick with your exercise plan. Keep your daily exercise card with you and follow it. It will be tough at first but will be easier as you stick with it.

In conclusion, I will leave you with this advice; in order to lose weight you must have a plan that includes both eating less, that is consuming less calories, and exercising routinely to take off the pounds that you have picked up over the years.

A good practice is to eat your bigger meals earlier and eat nothing after 7 p.m. and exercise after your last meal. This will increase your energy level and help you lose more calories as you sleep overnight.

I hope my example helps you as you take on your own battle with your weight.

May God be with you and bless you.

Richard Baud

DAILY EXERCISE CARD

Day of Week =

Time of Exercise
=

Type of Exercise
=

Amount of Time
Required to Exercise
=

I have found that how many calories I consume each day is the key to losing weight, I limit myself to a maximum of 7 times my current weight each day. Any more than this will cause me to gain weight. Therefore, here are some examples of how many calories a selection of foods contain:

Food	Serving Size (In grams)	Calories
6" Subway Club	256	320
6" Subway Turkey Breast	223	280
6" subway roast beef	223	290
6" subway ham	223	290
6" subway veggie delite	167	230
Saltine crackers	.75 ounces	230
English muffins	2 ounces	130
Plain waffles	1 ounce	84
Sweet roll	1 ounce	110
cheerios	½ cup	55
Raisin bran	1/3 cup	65
Colby cheese	2 table spoons	68
Cream cheese	2 tablespoons	101
jam	1 tablespoon	56
ketchup	1 tablespoon	15
mustard	1 tablespoon	10
Dill pickle	1 large	24
Pickled egg	1	135
Tarter sauce	1 tablespoon	70
Plain yogurt	4 ounces	69
brownie	2 inch square	112
Sponge cake	1 slice	187
Cheese cake	1 piece	309
Sugar cookie	1	98
Vanilla ice cream	½ cup	133
Apple pie	1 piece	277
Beef stew	1 cup	170

Cole slaw	½ cup	98
Ham salad	½ cup	270
Ham and cheese sandwich	1	352
Turkey sandwich	1	337
Steamed catfish	3 ounces	144
Fish sticks	2 ounces	112
Smoked halibut	3 ounces	153
Raw shad	4 ounces	223
Cooked tuna	3 ounces	130
apple	1	72
banana	1 large 8 inch	121
Sweet cherries	10	43
fig	1 large	47
Green grapes	½ cup	55
orange	1 large 3/16	86
peach	1 small	31
pear	1/2	50
strawberry	1 large	6
Beef jerky	0.7 ounces	81
Meat loaf	3.8 ounce slice	196
bacon	0.2 ounce	34
Pork hot dog	2.7 ounce	204
Cooked sausage	0.5 ounce	44
Chicken drumstick	3 ounce	174
Corn chips	1 ounce	145
Microwave popcorn/light butter	0.5 ounce	52
Soft pretzel	1 large	483
Chicken noodle soup	1 cup	80
Vegetable beef soup	1 cup	78
carrot	1 medium	25
celery	1 small stalk	8
cucumber	1-8 inch	45
Sweet ear corn	1 small ear	63

Snow peas	½ cup	13
spinach	3 ounces	20
Red tomato	1 medium	35
Burger king/angus steakburger	291 grams	690
Burger king big fish	250 grams	630
Vanilla milk shake	22 ounce	560
Pizza hut ham onions and mushrooms	1 slice	150
Brewed coffee	8 ounces	2
Unsweat tea	8 ounces	0
Apple cider	4 ounces	60
Orange juice	4 ounces	56
Whole milk	1 cup	146
Grape juice	4 ounces	71
Carrot juice	4 ounces	47
Hot cocoa with water	8 ounces	125
Rice milk	1 cup	144
Aquafina water	8 ounces	0

As I conclude this chapter I hope my examples of how to lose weight will help inspire you to do the same.

WALMART

When Sam Walton began Walmart, his big idea was to bring low prices to rural Americans, until he did, only urban communities had the ability to have a wide variety of products at good competitive prices. Of course, Sam's idea was amazing successful, not only did his (company) Walmart succeed but his ability to lead Walmart in a way that would push down the prices many Americans paid for their necessities has caused the standard of living to rise for millions of American around the country.

I want to give credit to Walmart's founder for establishing in his company Walmart some critical things. First thing:

He set the pace for Walmart to be very frugal and always looking for ways to keep cost down and in turn keeping the prices customers pay for those products down. Sam Walton deeply engrained this into all of us that worked for Walmart. And he was relentless at always keeping that competitive edge. I will give you an example of how Sam Walton thought. When Walmart was growing quickly in the late 1980's our Walmart buyers complained that the growth in the number of buyers and all of the bureaucracy that the growth brought with it had led to a shortage of phones and phone lines. The concern was brought to Sam Walton who considered the problem and after a while came back with this. Sam sent one-third of the buyers away from corporate headquarters to work as assistant managers to work in the Walmart stores, thus solving the problem of having too many people and to few phones.

Not the solution the buyers wanted but it solved the problem and helped keep the corporate headquarters from bloating and in turn kept cost down. Sam Walton was very competitive by nature and would be very aggressive at taking on any and all competitors that Walmart would face in the marketplace. As Walmart would come into a new market many local competitors would close simply because they did not adapt. Walmart brought with it lower prices and if a local retailer did not lower their prices they could not compete. Many local businesses made changes to their cost structures and product mix and were able to survive and even prosper.

Second thing:

That Sam Walton established in his company was giving the workers a pathway to move up within Walmart. At Walmart employees "Sam called us associates" could work hard and move up so much so that over 70% of all of the management teams around the country begin as hourly associates. This allowed thousands of normal hard-working people to live their own version of the American dream.

At Walmart this focus of folks moving up the company ladder kept our managements team real, when you supervise people doing the job that you once did, you can relate to them, and this leads to a very good rapport between hourly associates and the management that supervises them.

Third thing:

That Sam Walton established was basic respect. Sam treated people with respect, treating the average worker like we were important and have value within the company. Sam always took the time to talk to the associates, he listened to their concerns and was able to get great ideas from them. Sam always had a yellow notepad handy and would write down what the associates were telling him.

The success of Walmart has been well documented over the years. Walmart has not been perfect but has always had the ability to adapt to the changing retail environment and to keep focused on taking care of the customer. Having the customer as the focus keeps Walmart grounded.

One other thing about Walmart before I pivot to focus on my own

Walmart journey, even as Walmart became the number 1 retailer in the world and the biggest private company in America our Walmart executives were always running scared, scared of our competition overtaking us and scared of Walmart failing. This fear has been helpful in keeping all of Walmart focused on the customer and staying ahead of the competition.

I worked my way up in another retailer (Pamida) I started as a stock boy pushing shopping carts, cleaning restrooms, sweeping floors and doing anything that I was asked to do. I gradually worked my way up to sales associate, then department manager, then receiving manager, then to group manager. Pamida was my opportunity to start on my pathway to success. Then Walmart moved closer to my local town and I could see that Walmart held a lot more opportunities for me, so I hired on with Walmart.

I had given Pamida a two-week notice, they immediately fired me saying I was going to work for a competitor. I was to start at Walmart on January 12, 1981, they were kind enough to start me two weeks earlier on December 30, 1980, I could not afford to be out of work for two weeks.

So I begin my Walmart career on December 30, 1980 as a management trainee making $230 a week. I was 19 years old and excited about this opportunity. I had worked very hard to make my way up the ladder into management. I hoped Walmart would allow me the opportunity to continue to grow and succeed in life.

My training store was located in Benton, Illinois, the way the training plan worked was, you train for 16 weeks at the training store, then you were promoted to assistant manager and transferred to a different store. My first day as a trainee, my store manager Rick McClintock introduced me to all of the associates of the store "this is Richard Baud. He is our new management trainee. Richard will be with us for 16 weeks (my store manager went on to explain) that because Richard was sent here as a management trainee our store had to let two associates go to keep payroll in line." Christmas was over and it was normal to reduce staffing when sales declined after Christmas, but my arrival was given as the reason that two additional associates had to be let go. The management training program was supposed to have the trainee go around each part of the store and learn how that area worked, it did not work that way in practice.

My first day I was given a box cutter, a Walmart vest and told to help the Lawn and Garden center manager set up his garden center to the new spring lay out. I worked on this project for over a month.

My next assignment was in the stock room. I was shown how to use a two-wheeler and how to unload a Walmart truck, from that day until the end of my training I would be asked to help unload almost every Walmart truck that our store received. Gradually I was allowed to do some training in the store. I help set up the lamp modular layout and I was trying to knock a shelf in to place and it started a disaster. My shelf fell and knocked the next shelf down and continued like a domino until every lamp the store had on display fell and crashed into an awful mess. I was horrified and very embarrassed that I had created this very big and very public spectacle.

At this store and every other Walmart store that I was assigned to all had one thing in common, (Walmart associates) they are amazing, they work very hard and strive to take care of the customer. Many Walmart associates work lots of overtime, coming in early, staying late, doing whatever is needed to keep the store rolling.

I finished my sixteen weeks of training at Benton, Illinois. Basically cramming sixteen weeks of training into three or fours weeks of actual training. The vast majority of my time there I just helped where the management team told me to help. Mainly unloading trucks, stocking freight, and setting modulars around the store.

I have no complaints. I was learning about Walmart and was excited to get to my next store and become an assistant manager.

My first assignment as an assistant manager was at Walmart store 343, Taylorville, Illinois. My store manager was Bob Heiserer, this guy was awful. He would yell at his management team and his associates, belittling everyone in front of customers on the sales floor. I remember a couple of incidents that were just his normal way of dealing with people. One day a parakeet had escaped from his cage in the pet department, our pet department manager had grabbed a butterfly net from sporting goods and was running all over the store trying to catch the parakeet. The store manager saw the pet department manager chasing the bird and he picked up a phone and used the public announcement system (this was after the store was opened for business) to make the following announcement "Beth put the butterfly net down, stop chasing the silly bird and get your self back to work."

One day during a management meeting, one of my fellow assistant managers had picked up a call from an associate who was calling in to inform us that she would not be coming to work today because she had no clean clothes to wear. The store manager overheard the discussion and took the phone from the assistant manager and told the associate "Get your self into work or you are fired."

On another occasion during our management meeting, the store manager was mad because a customer had complained about not getting a refund on an item. The store manager told all management that if he gets one complaint over a refund from one more customer that he would take the keys from that assistant manager being complained about and that assistant manager could explain to the district manager why he lost his keys, and the district manager could decide whether to keep that assistant manager or not. So after that meeting, all of us assistant managers agreed to just give refunds to everyone whether it made sense or not.

Our store manager, Bob Heiserer would walk around the store, throwing merchandise off the counters if he thought the area was not neat enough, creating a very threatening environment for all that worked in that store.

The store manager wanted to get promoted to district manager so whenever he got word that a Walmart executive was headed to the store, he would work all the management in the store 16-hour days. And he would work hourly associates' overtime to get the store ready for that executive. This practice is fairly normal, but our store manager took it to a different level. He would rent uhaul trucks and load them up with anything around the store that he thought the Walmart executive would not like. Then he had associates drive the uhauls around town until the Walmart executive left the store.

Eventually our store manager got promoted to district manager, soon afterwards he got in a fist fight with his regional manager and was fired.

During my time at the Taylorville Walmart, Sam Walton came to the store for a store visit. This was my first time to meet him in person. Sam did what he always did when he visited a store, he would tour the store with all management then meet with the hourly associates, asking them how things were going and getting their ideas on how to improve things in the company. Then Sam Walton would have a meeting with all management. During this meeting Sam asked me why I left Pamida and joined Walmart. I explained to Sam that I had followed Walmart's move into Illinois, as Walmart moved into a town soon Pamida would close its doors. So I decided to move over to Walmart, I also told Mr. Sam that Pamida had a reputation for their buyers taking bribes. Mr. Sam then said that he hoped that I would find Walmart a more stable company and he said that he had started Walmart on basic Christian principles, including the Golden Rule. Mr. Sam mentioned that he was a Sunday School teacher at his church.

My next assistant manager assignment was to a new store, number 422 in Robinson, Illinois. Me and the rest of the management team all arrived before they had begun setting up the new store. This town Robinson, Illinois was the town that I was born in. Walmart was putting up lots of stores and had run into conflict with unions. The unions did not like the fact that Walmart was a non-union company, and the unions were trying to stop Walmart from setting up their stores without union workers and union rules.

At the store in Robinson, Illinois the unions had made it clear that they would stop the store from being set up with non-union workers. They intended to stop Walmart trucks from getting to the site of the new store. Walmart got word of what the union was planning, so it devised a plan to outwit the unions.

On Friday night, Walmart sent in a convoy of Walmart trucks loaded with all the fixtures that would be required to set up our store. In addition to the fixtures all arriving in one night, Walmart sent in a army of Walmart management and associates from all over that area to assist the new management team of our store to get all the Walmart trucks unloaded and get all the fixtures set up. So we worked nonstop from Friday night thru Sunday night to get the fixture trucks unloaded and get all the fixtures in the entire store set up and ready for merchandise to be delivered. Usually this process took two or more weeks.

This effort stopped the union from interfering with Walmart's efforts to get this store set up. Walmart used the same tactic in towns all over Illinois.

During my time as assistant manager I worked in six different stores as a regular assistant manager. And I was also sent to 13 different stores from Indiana to Florida to help new stores set their stores up which included:

1. Setting up fixtures
2. Filling the store with merchandise
3. Hiring and training new associates to be ready to take care of customers and run the business.

My last assignment as assistant manager was at store No. 492 at Vincennes, Indiana. My district manager, Freddy Wesson had promised me that if I went to this store and helped get it fixed (because it was being ran poorly) that he would see to it that I got promoted to store manager within the next six months. So I was sent to the store on a Thursday and I met with the store manager Gary Cloniger. After talking to Gary for a few minutes we walked around the store looking at where the problems were and discussed what was needed to correct those problems. A few minutes later Gary told me that he was going to be off for a four-day weekend and that I was in charge of the store. I did not know the management or the associates, but I did know Walmart and quickly started correcting the problems. I mentioned that Gary left Thursday morning, I was told later by some associates that the associates schedule for the next week had not been completed. The schedules were supposed to be completed three weeks early, so that the associated could plan out their lives around the store's schedules. So my first day at that store I stayed until the early hours of the next morning preparing the associates schedules for the next week that started on Saturday. This is how my first day at that store went. Over the next six months I got to know the management and associates of that store, and we worked together to correct the problems the store had. Meanwhile the store manager did very little to help, he mainly stayed in his office.

Then on a Monday morning the local bank called and said that the entire weekend cash deposits were missing. This caused panic all over Walmart's chain of command and the local police were called in to help investigate. Long story short, the store manager Gary Cloniger had took the deposits Sunday evening and was supposed to drop them off at the bank. Instead, he had forgot to drop them off at the bank and left the money in his corvette. Gary kept saying that he knew nothing about where the deposits were, then miraculously they appeared in the banks overnight deposits. Gary would be removed from his position of store manager soon after this incident. I finished my six months at store 492, ending my time as assistant manager. I can tell you that in every one of the 20 stores I was involved in as assistant manager, there was always incredible hard working associates and management that did their job with pride and always acted like a family working as a team to take care of their customers.

On June 24, 1985, I became the store manager of Walmart No. 736, Russellville, Ky. This store was a 44,000 sq. foot store, it was a Big K acquisition store. The store started as a Big K store (not Kmart). In 1981 Walmart bought out the Big K company and converted the stores into Walmart stores. My new store was technically a Walmart store but had a lot of old Big K associates that were operating just like they did when Big K operated the store, the fixtures were held together by baling wire, so this store would prove to be very challenging to manage.

My new district manager, Bill Barlar checked me into the store on a Monday, then he was arrested for a DUI and was sentenced to do 30 days in what they called a drunk tank. Designed to help the inmate dry out from their dependence of alcohol. So it would be over a month before I would see any Walmart executives. No problem even though I was only 24 years old, my experiences from the last four and a half years taught me all I needed to know about how to manage a Walmart store. Walmart had two huge manuals on how the company expected it stores to be managed. I used those manuals to show the associates of that store (many who were old Big K employees) how to do stuff the Walmart way. This was not at all popular with the old crowd, I will expand on this. Right before I came to that store there had been a big criminal case solved involving over 20 of the Big K associates, apparently one of the assistant managers had hired a personnel manager and between the two of them they hired a den of thieves that robbed the store blind. When the case was over the police found over $250,000 of stolen property stored in a local storage rental place. Walmart of course fired all involved and charged many with criminal offensives.

Obviously this store did not observe many of the policies designed to keep honest associates honest and keep people with bad intentions from having opportunities to steal. In addition the store had loose operating standards one example was the padlocks on the doors had combination locks with the combinations written on the back of the lock (in case you forget the combination). The store had a total of 77 associates when I arrived, this included 30 associates who were either department managers, office associates or some kind of support member. These 30 associates ran the store while doing very little physical work, their days consisted mainly of having meetings in the lounge, where they would drink coffee, smoke and talk bad about their management team and the other 47 associates who actually did the physical work in the store. This group of 30 associates had agreed (before I even arrived at the store) to not cooperate with the new store manager, and they would continue doing things the way they were used to doing them. This group resisted everything I tried to accomplish in the store, no problem I can be very determined and over the next six months I changed the store. I had to terminate 26 associates out of the 77 associates that were there when I arrived, I hired new associates and trained them how Walmart wanted things done. Also I was able to convert many of the former Big K associates into really good Walmart associates even though the first six months was very very tough, this store would grow and be a very good Walmart store.

I will complete my story about store 736 with a couple of incidents that happened while I was there.

The first incident:

One of my assistant managers Mike Plankars, who was a military veteran who had managed a supply depot with over one billon dollars in assets, called our district manager "Bill". Now Bill Barlar was used to being call Mr. Barlar, so he was really mad about the lack of respect and demanded I discipline Mike Plankars, so I complied and completed the formal disciplinary action, soon afterwards Mr. Walton who was usually referred to (as Mr. Sam or Mr. Walton) sent out a memo to all Walmart executives and every store associate around the company, simply stating that our company would drop the formality of referring to Walmart executives and Walmart management as Mr. or Mrs., and call everyone by their first name. Of course the next time Bill Barlar arrived in our store, Mike Plankars rushed to greet him and say "Good morning Bill." It always amazes me as to how things change and how some folks fight the change and others embrace it.

The second incident:

Was when Sam Walton visited my store, Sam would fly his small corporate plane into local airports and call the store and have someone come and pick him up from the airport and drive him to the local Walmart store. When Sam Walton landed at the Russellville, Ky. airport he found that it was basically just a landing strip used by local farmers to dust their crops. There was no one at the airport (this was before cell phones) so Sam Walton, the richest man in America, had to hitch hike from the airport to my store. A local farmer gave him a ride in an old pickup truck.

Sam Walton visited my store and found the store to be in great shape and complimented my associates for doing such a great job. This was the same store that barely resembled a Walmart store just two years earlier, it just proves that with a group of people working together you can accomplish almost anything. While he was visiting privately with me, Sam invited me to come to Walmart headquarters and interview to be become a buyer, when Sam Walton left my store, we drove him back to the airport. Sam Walton was proud that he had to hitch hike to get to my store.

I did go to Walmart headquarters to interview to be a buyer, but during the interview I was told that I would be working in an office where my next three levels of supervision would all be within a few yards of me. I never really liked to be supervised in the first place, so I thanked them for the offer and returned to where I was comfortable, my store. Before I left store 736 my store would relocate to the other side of Russellville and be twice as big and a brand new up to date Walmart store. Me and my associates where really proud of our new store. I was promoted to a bigger store soon afterwards where my journey with Walmart would continue. As with all the Walmart's I was part of, Russellville, Ky's Walmart had awesome associates. Walmart has the good fortune to have such good quality people that make up their workforce.

My next store that I would manage was Walmart store No. 673. This store was located on Wilma Rudolph Blvd. across from Governors Square Mall, in Clarksville, Tn. This store was larger than my Russellville, Ky. store and had a bigger population base, which meant that the store was busier than store 736. Being a bigger town made it more difficult to keep good quality associates. I quickly learned to appreciate one group of associates that the store had. Clarksville, Tn. is a military town with Ft. Campbell based nearby, so my new store employed a significant number of military spouses, these associates were top notch. They would transfer to a nearby Walmart when their spouse would transfer to a new military base. These associates were already trained and fit in very quickly, adding stability to my new store. If you own or manage a business close to a military base, I highly recommend that you seek out the spouses of the soldiers for employment.

It was at this store that I was witnessed to an amazing scene, my district manager had called for a district meeting at the hotel across from my store. These meetings were routine and gave the district manager a way to share information with all of that district's store managers at one time. Two things happened at this meeting that would lead to a wild Walmart experience. First, Bill Barlar and most of the store managers smoked and even though smoking at Walmart meetings had been banned recently by our founder Sam Walton, our district manager lit up his cigarette, so the store managers that smoked also lit up their cigarettes. Soon smoke filled the room and it looked like a pool hall instead of a Walmart meeting. The second thing that happened at that meeting was that the district manager, Bill Barlar was complaining that our district had way too many resident assistant managers. This just meant that the assistant manager had been promoted at the local Walmart and would not be able to transfer to other nearby Walmart's, making it difficult for the district manager to keep his high turnover stores staffed with quality assistant managers. Then it happened, Sam Walton had arrived unexpectantly at my store. My assistant manager immediately called me (not so easy back then, no cell phones), so he called the front desk at the hotel from my store's landline phone. I answered the phone to be told that my assistant manager had met Sam Walton and explained that I was across the street at a district meeting. Sam Walton said, "No problem, I will go and join the district meeting." So Sam Walton was on his way to the district meeting, it was a very quick trip, literally across the street. So I got off the phone and located my boss, Bill Barlar and informed him that Sam Walton was on his way.

Bill Barlar literally ran to the meeting room and shouted to the store managers to get rid of their cigarettes!!!!!! In a matter of three minutes all cigarettes were put out and everyone started opening all the windows in the meeting room trying to fan the smoke out of the room. It was a wild scene, grown men running around trying to hide the fact that they had been smoking.

Soon Sam Walton entered the hotel lobby, Bill Barlar met him there and tried to stall him as long as possible to allow the smoke to clear from the room. Sam soon entered the meeting room which was still very smoky. He looked around and took a big whiff and just smiled, never saying a word about the smoky smell. Bill Barlar and the store managers that had been smoking all looked like children that had been caught with their hands in a cookie jar.

Sam Walton then met with our district manager and all of us store managers. Sam touched base on a lot of issues and as always asked for feed back from us on current issues concerning the company.

Then Sam looked at Bill Barlar and said, "I want to thank you for having the highest percentage of resident assistant managers in the company." Sam went on to explain how important the resident assistant manager position was and how it helped keep stability in a store. And if you remember Bill Barlar had been complaining to us store managers about having too many resident assistant managers in our district. All of a sudden Bill Barlar became the biggest supporter of the resident assistant manager program. Telling Sam Walton how proud he was to have that many resident assistant managers in that district. After Sam Walton left the meeting Bill Barlar said, "Forget what I said earlier, we will be adding resident assistant managers in my district."

This was one of the funniest days that I had during my career at Walmart. It falls under the heading you could not believe it unless you were there.

At that Clarksville Walmart I also witnessed one of the saddest experiences of my Walmart career. On a busy Saturday afternoon, I got a message that a customer had a serious medical issue in our greeting card department. Me and my management team rushed over to see what was going on, a customer, a gentleman in his 70's just had a massive heart attack and died and fell over into the greeting cards. This gentleman had been a professor at a college in Illinois. He had retired after 50 years of service literally the day before. The professor and his wife had left Illinois for a long vacation. They had merely stopped at my store to pick up a few things, planning to continue their journey later. Talking to the professor's wife they never took vacations and were planning on catching up since her husband had retired. The professor's wife could not drive, so there she was hundreds of miles away from home. Her husband of over 50 years dying so suddenly and she could not drive. Their family was called and would come to take care of their mom and make arrangements for their dad. In the meantime, our associates and management kicked into action. We secured a hotel room for her, and we had associates to volunteer to cook her food for every meal. And also, we had associates that would take turns staying with her, so she didn't have to be alone. This was a tragic event, but I was so proud of how our team came together to assist this lady in her time of need. This type of genuine caring is very common among Walmart associates.

I would soon be off to my next store manager assignment.

My next store to manage was Walmart store no. 1825, Manassas, Virginia. This town was in the middle of lots of civil war battles, the most famous was The Battle of Bull Run. When I arrived in Manassas, I found out that this store had a bad history itself. This store was the first Walmart that was built in the eastern part of the United States, and the executives that planned the store had vastly underestimated some key factors. First, the sales were a lot higher than expected. Second, since Manassas was the furthest Walmart east, Walmart had not correctly planned how to get the store replenished. Adding these two factors together the shelves were virtually empty for weeks after the store opened. The store was so bad that the current CEO of Walmart complained in an interview (that had nationwide readership) about the Manassas store, saying that it was an example of how not to open a store in a new part of the country.

During my first visit from the regional vice president, Larry Williams, Larry told me that he was almost fired over the conditions of the Manassas store (before I got there). This was a tough store and would take a while to correct the problems. Luckily, we had a core of good associates that were willing to work hard, including lots of overtime to do their part to turn the store around. When I arrived, the store was understaffed to a point that we had to add a second personal manager to just hire new associates. We set up a conference room at the motel across from Walmart and we would hire 30 or more new Walmart associates a month until about six months later we finally had enough associates to properly staff the store. Once we were staffed the store turned around and started to look and feel like a good Walmart store. The store remained a very visible Walmart because of how it opened, so we had lots of executive visits to the store. Manassas had an airport where a corporate jet could land and refuel without any additional fees. This was the only airport in the entire area around Washington, D.C. that did not charge any additional fees. So all Walmart executives that wanted to come to the Washington, D.C. area would land their corporate jet at the Manassas airport, then drive to the Walmart store they wanted to see. So many of the Walmart executives would find time to visit my store. I would have to pick them up at the Manassas airport and bring them to my store. During one of the many times I was at that airport,

I had a big surprise. I went to the men's room to visit the urinal, when all of a sudden four well-armed men busted into the men's room and looked at every stall and checked out the rest of the restroom making sure that it was safe for then former President George Bush to use the urinal. So there I was using the urinal with four secret service agents standing at attention in the room. Looking out for Mr. Bush who used the urinal next to the one I was using. Mr. Bush told me that he was sorry to make such a commotion in the restroom. I told Mr. Bush that it was not a problem and I told him that I had voted for him and was sorry that he had lost. Mr. Bush said that he had been proud to serve and looking forward to returning to Texas. Life in Manassas was always interesting, and that store would be the hardest store to manage. I had to work 70-80 hours a week just to keep the store running smooth. Manassas, Virginia was located outside of Washington, D.C. about 45 minutes from the White House, so we would have a steady stream of federal government bureaucrats visit my store to make sure that we were up to current government regulations. Walmart always tried to follow all laws and regulations, but it was a challenge to have the regulators in the store all the time.

One of the most bizarre situations came up at this store. We had an associate name Bob that was a special needs individual. Bob had some issues but we hired him to do simple tasks, mainly throwing cardboard into the cardboard baler. Bob was very dependable and worked hard at his job. Bob always wore a denim shirt and had a denim backpack that he would use to carry his lunch, etc. Bob lived several blocks from the Walmart store and would walk everyday to work. One day an officer came into the store and asked to see the store manager. I asked what I could do for him, and he said, "we have one of your employees named Bob, he robbed the bank a couple of blocks from the store." Reportedly the bank had just been robbed and the bank teller had identified Bob as the bank robber. I was shocked, surely Bob would not rob a bank. The officer was only telling me about the bank robbery and Bob being identified as the robber as a courtesy to me. I told the officer that I could not imagine Bob doing this. I worked with my personnel manager and my management team to do our own investigation. Luckily we still used a time clock to punch in and out, to record the time the associates worked so they would be paid correctly. As it turned out Bob was still on the clock at the time the bank was robbed. Bob had just left Walmart a few minutes after the bank was robbed and walked home like he did everyday in front of that bank. The bank was robbed, and the police immediately started looking for the subject that was wearing a denim shirt and denim backpack. The police found Bob a couple of blocks from the bank. Bob's description matched the description that the bank teller had given the police, they took Bob to the bank and the teller identified Bob as the bank robber. When we discovered that the timeline was not right and Bob could not be in two places at one time, the police restarted their search for the real bank robber and quickly found the real bank robber and Bob was released. If it had been for the time clock evidence, Bob had a big chance of going to prison for a crime he did not commit (very scary).

Interesting people at Walmart no. 1825: My very best assistant manager Dung Tran. Dung was a Vietnamese man who had spent 444 days on a boat and at a refugee camp when he escaped from Viet Nam after the Viet Nam war had ended. Dung's father was an officer in the south Vietnamese military, and when the war was over Dung's father was sent to a reeducation camp and Dung and his family would suffer at the hands of the Vietnamese government, including not being able to secure a job. So Dung fled with many others as soon as he could. Dung would find his way to Manassas, Virginia and he was working at the Manassas Walmart when I arrived at that store. Dung was working on third shift as a stocker, he worked so hard and put everything into his job, soon I was able to promote him to third shift assistant manager. Dung was the very best assistant manager I've ever had at any Walmart. He worked hard and had those working for him work just as hard, Dung could not communicate in English very well but made up for that difficulty by his effort level. Before I left the Manassas store, Dung had been promoted to store manager in Delaware (what a success story.)

Another awesome Associate, was a gentleman named Wayne Zitzke,

Wayne was an older fellow who had an interesting life before Walmart, that included being a prison guard at the prison where Charles Manson was being Imprisoned.

Wayne was a people greeter for the Manassas Walmart, when I arrived at the store.

Wayne told me about a great experience that he had just had, Wayne worked with an organization from Washington DC, he had volunteered to take an underprivileged child with him on a fishing trip. Wayne said that the child had never been fishing before and this child had a great day of fishing with Wayne, Wayne could not stop talking about this awesome experience.

Soon Wayne talked me into making it into a store project (to take local children fishing)Wayne would work with our vendors to get them to contribute fishing supplies, including Fishing rods, tackle boxes, coolers snacks drinks etc and we also did car washes, bake sales and community wide craft sales (on Walmart's parking lot) to raise money to support the fishing trip.

The first fishing trip that we did had only a few children, but would eventually grow into a massive annual event that would raise over $30000 a year and take hundreds of our local children to a local lake.

Our Walmart supplied a mentor with each child and between what the vendors donated and what our store would raise in funds, we were able to supply each child with their own fishing rod and fishing supplies and everything that the children needed for the fishing trip, all of this happened because of the experience Wayne had with one Child that experienced fishing for the first time.

Wayne would start out every one of our planning meetings with the same phrase (It is for the children) Wayne Zitzke made a difference in lots of childrens lives by his efforts to give those wonderful little children the experience of fishing.

Walmart#1825 Manassas Virginia was a great experience for me, I appreciate all of the Awesome Associates that I had the privilege of working with.

Now it was time for me to move on to my next Walmart Store.

Walmart chapter 5

My next Walmart store to manage was Walmart store #192 in Columbia Tennessee.

In chapter 3 of this book I went into detail about how me and my family went from Manassas Virginia to Columbia Tennessee, the story of how God allowed so many things to happen to Rip us out of Manassas Virginia and replant us in Columbia Tennessee was so remarkable that there was no doubt in my mind that God had plans for me and my family in Columbia Tennessee.

I officially started at the Columbia Walmart on 5-1-1998, I had accepted Jesus as my personal Savior on 12-15-1996 and had gradually learned to live by faith.

Now after the experience of seeing God move so clearly in my life I knew that God had a plan for my life that included the Columbia Walmart and the Town of Columbia Tennessee, so unlike previous Walmart stores that I had managed this Walmart had something special, God had put me here and I needed to act like it. So at this Walmart I would no longer Solely rely on my own talents and abilities, I started to pray each day and ask God to protect me in my job at Walmart and I asked God to Help me make decisions that would be pleasing to him.

The Columbia Walmart was a division one Store which means that it was not a grocery store yet, this store was the same size as my store in Manassas, so it was very easy to adjust to.

Columbia Tennessee was a town of 37000 people and was in the middle of Maury County with a population of 67000 people.

Columbia's claim to fame is Mule Day, for over 200 years Columbia has celebrated mules including a Parade which has over 100000 Attendees, the entire week preceding the Parade the town has Events including a liar's contest and booths from local Businesses and individuals selling food drink and all kinds of knickknacks.

Columbia is mainly a bedroom community with a good amount of its citizens commuting to Nashville Tennessee for work, there are also factories scattered around this area that include the General Motors plant in Spring Hill Tennessee and the Maury regional hospital and related medical service facilities that provide the community with jobs.

For the most part these jobs did not pay well except for the General Motors plant in Spring Hill. Hourly Wages in Franklin Tennessee and Nashville Tennessee were usually $1 to $2 higher so many Maury County residents would choose to make the 30-60 minute commute to get the additional wages.

This fact has been a drain on the available labor pool, making it difficult to maintain a steady work force at my Columbia Walmart, we always had to work hard to keep our good employees.

When I first arrived at the Columbia Walmart, I noticed right away that the store was run down looking, lots of fix up and clean up projects had to be completed before the store would be up to the standards that Walmart required.

But the store had a core of very good Associates so it did not take long to correct the problem areas. Meanwhile at home my youngest Two children were having trouble adjusting to their new schools. We had left Virginia with several weeks left in the current school year, but since Tennessee starts their school year earlier my children had only two weeks left in their new classes, the transition to a new school all new classes and no friends was just awful for them, every morning for the entire two weeks they cried and were (reluctant to say the least) to go to school, me and Ramona agreed that we would not leave Columbia until all of our kids were done with school so that our kids would not have to go thru that kind of trauma ever again switching schools.

Well they made it through those awful two weeks and made some new friends and got out of school in early May while their former classmates in Virginia still had another month in school.

My youngest son Samuel came home from school one day during those two weeks repeating a story that he was told, the story was about my predecessor (the previous store manager of the Columbia Tennessee Walmart store) he had been removed from his position as store manager for dating one of his Assistant managers.

This was a true story but it seemed odd to me that 5th graders would know what happened at their local Walmart store, so word gets around quickly in Columbia Tennessee.

My Walmart in Columbia Tennessee is located in the middle of town and is several miles off of the interstate so we did not receive a lot of visits from Walmart Executives

The Executives like to go down the interstate and visit lots of Walmart stores as they go, so a Walmart located off the beaten path would not get very many Executive visits.

The Columbia Walmart also in an odd geographic area which meant that we would constantly shift from belonging to one District one year and shift to a different one the next year.

So in my 22 years as the store manager I had a lot of different District managers some were good others were not so good but they rarely made a difference in my store.

My management team and Associates took pride in keeping the store in good shape and focused on taking care of our Customers, my management style was to provide our Associates with the resources they needed to do their jobs provide good direction and establish priorities for the store based on what Walmart Corporation expected then get out of their way and let them get it done, I always encouraged our Associates to have a good time while working I figured that if you spent 1/3 of your time at work you should be able to be a human being not a machine as store manager I would spend most of my time dealing with poor performers and hiring new Associates to replace them.

My biggest delight as a Walmart store manager was watching Walmart Associates and our Management team grow and take on new positions and more responsibility, the Columbia Walmart has seen a large number of hourly Associates promoted to the Management team and lots of our Management team move into higher roles, at one time the Store managers for the Spring Hill, Lewisburg, Hohenwald, Shelbyville, Lawrenceville, Lebanon, and two of the Murfreesboro stores all were trained by our Columbia Associates and management team. Meanwhile when my family moved to Columbia we started to look for a good local Church to attend we went to every Baptist Church in Columbia some twice. At some point we went to Northside Baptist Church, I can tell you that this Church is special you can feel the Holy

Spirit moving and the Congregation made my family feel welcome, but we were not convinced on the first visit, so we returned for a second visit. The Preacher said one sentence that we had heard our last Preacher say every week Pastor Rushing said (We must keep the main thing the main thing) meaning that the focus of the Church is Leading people to Jesus. At that moment me and Ramona knew that God had led us to this Church.

Within a few months the Sunday school director and his family moved out of town and our Pastor asked me to be the Sunday school director remember I had only been saved less than 2 years and I had no clue of what a Sunday school director even does I talked it over with Ramona and Prayed on it and felt the Lord telling me to do it, so I accepted the position and I continued in that role for 10 years. I realize now that Northside Baptist Church was one of the reasons that God had led my family to Columbia Tennessee.

Northside Baptist Church and the wonderful people of that Church would be a vital part of my family's lives.

I thank God for his amazing blessings, I have three families, My immediate family, my Church family and my Walmart family all have came together to create a wonderful life for me.

Back to Walmart

On 3-20-2002 we opened our brand new Walmart supercenter in Columbia Tennessee, the day we opened the store we had 636 hourly Associates on the payroll, we had a very good hourly Associate team and a very good Management team, so this new Supercenter was awesome from day one. The first year we did $106 million in sales and we would continue doing over $100 million in sales every year for over 20 years this amount of sales volume takes a lot of hard work and team work to keep the shelves stocked and customers taken care of properly, even though me nor my team was perfect we managed to provide a great store for our community and our team would go all over the middle part of Tennessee assisting other Walmart stores that needed help for various reasons.

Our store was recognized for its performance in 2012 we received two awards

- Region 15 Supercenter of the year (the best of over 100 other Walmarts)
- MRD (divisional) Supercenter of the year (the best of over 600 other Walmarts)

A copy of both awards are attached.

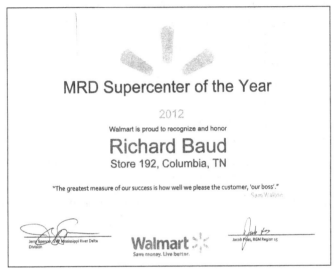

MRD Supercenter of the Year

2012

Walmart is proud to recognize and honor

Richard Baud

Store 192, Columbia, TN

"The greatest measure of our success is how well we please the customer, 'our boss'."
Sam Walton

Jerry Spencer, SVP Mississippi River Delta Division

Walmart ☀
Save money. Live better.

Jacob Fras, RGM Region 15

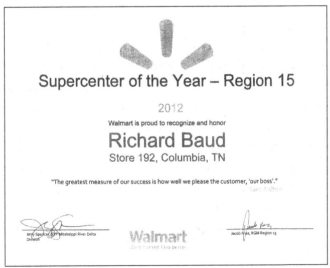

Supercenter of the Year – Region 15

2012

Walmart is proud to recognize and honor

Richard Baud

Store 192, Columbia, TN

"The greatest measure of our success is how well we please the customer, 'our boss'."
Sam Walton

Jerry Spencer, SVP Mississippi River Delta Division

Walmart
Save money. Live better.

Jacob Fras, RGM Region 15

The Columbia Tennessee Walmart store # 192 has been blessed with amazing Associates, I want to recognize some of the best, this group is in no way complete (there are many many more) but will give you an idea of who the people are behind the Walmart vests, I will start off with Martha Lentz who worked with us for nearly 30 years Martha managed the front end of our store like a General Commanding her troops treating her people with respect but expecting her folks to do their jobs well and provide great customer service.

Next is Lana Almacher, Lana managed our third shift operation for years responsible for stocking the store Lana was a petite lady that had the spirit of a roaring Lion she managed her group of Associates so well that the nights that Lana was off whoever took charge of the third shift operation those nights could never match the results that Lana achieved with the same Associates.

Next to recognize is Ricky Byrd, Ricky managed our electronics Department for 30 years keeping up with all the technology and managing our highest sales volume Department in our store keeping the shrink (theft and paperwork) to a level unparalleled in our District, Ricky maintained his area to a high level and was so knowledgeable that Customers would ask for him by name.

Next to recognize is Jerry Braden, Jerry was head of of our loss prevention/Security Department for many years Jerry had a knack for spotting shoplifters. For many years Jerry would catch over 500 shoplifters a year, Jerry had many scary situations including being shot at and threatened with a knife, Fortunately Jerry was always the Victor keeping our Columbia Police Department very busy, while Jerry managed Security our store was able to keep our retail Shrinkage (including theft) to very low levels helping maintain our Stores profit.

Next to recognize is Betsy Fly, Betsy managed our Domestics Department when we were in the old store (Where Belks is located now) also Betsy has managed several other Departments including Dairy/frozen and the Hardware Department, Betsy had stage 4 Cancer and beat it and Betsy continues to be one of the hardest working Associates in the store.

Next to recognize is Brenda Blatt, Brenda at an age that many consider retiring still can outwork any 20 year old and Brenda lets them know it.

Next to recognize is Doris Claude, Doris managed one of the toughest areas in the store our Deli Department (this area is hot and greasy and has very demanding Customers) Doris took pride in her area and demanded that those that worked under her supervision did the same.

Next to recognize is Evelyn Drewett, Evelyn is a tornado she works so quickly and so hard that normally two Associates could not put out the work that Evelyn does, Evelyn has held many positions in the store and has excelled in every one of them.

Next to recognize is Tiffany Love, Tiffany has held many positions in the store and has a reputation for being a tough Leader who cares about those that she supervises, Tiffany has created many top quality Associates that go on to important positions in the store.

Next to recognize is Chris Lonas, Chris started out in our layaway Department and made his way into the Vision Center where he rose to the position of Vision Center Manager, Chris has helped teach and train Associates who are now on their way to Major Professional positions in the Vision Center.

Next to recognize is Valerie Logan, Valerie has held lots of positions in our store including Customer service Manager where Valerie ran a tight ship managing over 100 cashiers. Valerie would not allow the Customers to wait at the checkouts sometimes Valerie would have to show out to make it happen but she did make it happen, Valerie went on to go into management and has helped our store and other area Walmart stores in Management roles.

Next to recognize is Parish Phelps, Parish was a third shift stocker when I arrived at the Columbia Walmart, he was the first person that I promoted to management in this store, Parish has held lots of management positions in our store and in each of those positions Parish treated his Associates with care and always had the Associate's interest in mind.

Next to recognize is Kayla Cole, Kayla started as a third shift Stocker working her way into management Kayla first went to the Murfreesboro Walmart (the Walmart next to MTSU) where she excelled running their third shift operation, after her time was up at that store (when you get promoted into management you had to stay at your first management position for 18 months before being eligible to transfer to a different Walmart store) Kayla returned to our store first as e-commerce / pickup manager where she lead a large group of Associates in a very fast paced and difficult part of the Store, Kayla was recognized by our regional Vice President during an executive visit to our store for having managed a great Department and for having a Bright future at Walmart, during another Walmart restructuring Kayla was put in charge of the entire third shift operation, putting Kayla back on third shift that Kayla loves.

Next to recognize is Diane Upchurch, Diane has worked in many positions in the store including people greeter, where Diane once hugged a customer (as Diane is prone to do) the elderly customer cried telling Diane that she was the first person to hug her in months, wherever Diane worked in the store she made a personal connection with everyone that she worked with.

Next to recognize is Ann Travis, Ann was a cashier for many years, while in this role Ann made sure that anyone who was sick or had a death in the family received a greeting card, signed by many Walmart Associates, Ann made many Associations feel important and cared for, Truly doing the Lord's work.

The final Associate on this list of awesome associates that I need to recognize is Danielle Brown, Danielle started with Walmart in 1996 and has impacted many areas of the store Danielle managed the layaway Department for years teaching and training new Associates each year, Danielle excelled in this position running one of the best layaway Departments in our Region.

When Danielle's daughter was born pre-mature and spent time in the Prenatal unit at Vanderbilt Children's Hospital in Nashville Tennessee, Danielle saw how much good that Children's hospital did and she became the leader in our store in support of the Children's Miracle

Network Campaign (raising money to help support the Vanderbilt Children's Hospital) with Danielle's leadership our store became a leader in our part of Tennessee in the amount of money raised for this important cause (one year raising over $60000) Danielle would inspire reluctant cashiers and other Associates to ask Customers for support, letting them know how much good it does for local Children.

Danielle would later become involved in our personnel and training Department where she was a caring person for Associates in need of support to go to. Danielle would help Associates get the assistance that they needed regardless of how much time or effort it required. Danielle never let a child especially a baby of an Associate leave the personnel office without a big hug.

Whatever job position Danielle had, she worked hard and quickly to get the job done.

I would ask Danielle for advice on many people issues that came up over the years Danielle would always be a check on me if I was getting ready to make a bad decision.

As with many positions at Walmart the Personnel manager position would be changed Walmart went from a full time Personnel manager and a full time Training co-ordinator down to only one job position combining both of the previous positions into one job position.

Walmart did what is now the Corporations "go to" procedure, they change the job description and make existing Associates apply for a job position that they had previously held, this is a way they have established in order to get people that match the Corporate philosophy and priorities and eliminate people that do not.

As the Company rolled out this new Personnel manager position it had such a complicated process to select who would get this position including group interviews designed to make it very difficult for existing Associates to make it thru the process.

Thereby eliminating most of the existing personnel managers and training co-ordinations from getting the new personnel managers position.

Danielle applied for this position and was not chosen because "she was too close to the Associates in our store" Danielle was offered the personnel manager role in other Walmart stores, but she did not want to work at other Walmarts so she did not accept those offers.

When I as the store manager challenged the decision on not offering the personnel manager position in my store to Danielle I was told by the market manager (my immediate supervisor) that the decision was made by the Regional Vice President.

Of course I then used Walmart's open door policy and asked the Regional Vice President about the decision He told me that the Market manager had made the decision and the decision was his to make, after exhausting all avenues with the Walmart bureaucracy, I and many of our Associates and our management team turned to prayer asking God to intervene.

God is good, soon a couple of amazing things happened.

First the person who had been selected to be Columbia's personnel manager turned down the position. Second the position was re-opened and Danielle was allowed to be considered for the position. (this was a good step but remember that Danielle had been "considered" for the position before.

Third the Market manager asked me what we should do about the position, of course I told the market manager to do what he should have done in the first place give the position (that Danielle was uniquely qualified for) to Danielle.

Fourth the market manager agreed and sent the recommendation to the Regional Vice President who approved offering the position to Danielle.

Without a doubt God had intervened and fixed the situation in such a striking manner.

Danielle accepted the position and has done a great job at it like she did at every other job position she has had at Walmart.

While I am discussing Danielle Brown, I have to tell you about some of her (sayings)

Danielle is very smart but sometimes goes into what I call Daniellism's as she expresses herself in the spoken word.

Here are some of her Daniellism's.

1. I got a hold to (meaning I talked to)
2. I had to spoke up (meaning I had to speak up)

3. I got on my thinking face (I still don't know what that means)
4. You are such a lie (meaning you are such a liar)
5. don't get no smack with me (meaning don't talk smack to me)
6. people are stressing me up (meaning people are stressing me out)
7. I am usually the one that un does stuff (meaning that she fixes stuff that others mess up)
8. I learn't (meaning I found out)
9. you do the most least (I still don't know what that means)
10. I hadn't said any much (I still don't know what that means)
11. more higher (meaning more than)
12. low easy Anna (meaning Louisiana)
13. if she ever blurbs it out take it and go (meaning if she quits let her)

These sayings (plus many many others) have kept me and many others entertained for years. Thank you Danielle!!!!!

The following are copies of several newsletters that were given to our Walmart Associates over the years.

These newsletters will give you an idea of what was happening in the store over the years.

The Wal-Mart Smiley Town News
December 1999
Volume 1 Issue 6

A Note From Richard.

Dear Wal-Mart Associates,

While Christmas is drawing near, we at Wal-Mart are busy unloading trucks, stocking shelves, ringing up customers and helping shoppers in the store. I would like to take a moment to reflect upon the true meaning of Christmas, and to share an experience that happened to me at a Wal-Mart that changed my life.

The reason for the season is Jesus Christ. Almost 2000 years ago Jesus Christ was born, sent by God to be a Savior to all mankind. I think on his birthday that it is only right to remember the great sacrifice of his death by crucifixion, and the following resurrection. He did this all for our sakes, so that anyone who calls on his name can be saved and have eternal everlasting life. In relation to this, I will tell you of a personal experience, and since Wal-Mart has been a very important part of my life for a long time, it is only fitting that it occurred at Wal-Mart.

It was a busy Friday in the middle of December 1996. While I was the Store Manager of the Wal-Mart in Manassa, Virginia, one of our Department Managers, Lennette Hutt, gave me a poem entitled, "Twas The Night Before Jesus Came." As I read this poem I was crushed. For the first time in my life I realized that I would never see Jesus or go to Heaven because I was not saved.

The next two days Jesus worked on me. I felt his presence and I was convicted and I knew that I needed to be saved. That Sunday, December 15, 1996, as our preacher gave the invitation, I walked to the front of the church and asked Jesus to forgive me for my sins, and I gave my life to Jesus! That same day I was baptized, and am proud to say that my children have all been saved and now I look forward to the day Jesus will return.

May God Bless You All,
Richard Baud
12/15/99

TWAS THE NIGHT BEFORE JESUS CAME

Twas the night before Jesus came and all through the house,
Not a creature was praying, not one in the house.
Their Bibles were lain on the shelf without care,
In hopes that Jesus would not come there.

The children were dressing to crawl into bed,
Not once ever kneeling or bowing a head.
And Mom in the rocker with Baby on her lap,
Was watching the Late Show while I took a nap.

When out of the East there arose such a clatter,
I sprang to my feet to see what was the matter.
Away to the window I flew like a flash!
Tore open the shutters and threw up the sash!

When what to my wondering eyes should appear,
But angels proclaiming that Jesus was here!
With a light like the sun sending forth a bright ray,
I knew in a moment this must be the day.

The light of his face made me cover my heard,
It was Jesus returning just like he said.
And though I possessed worldly wisdom and wealth,
I cried when I saw him in spite of myself.

In The Book of Life which he held in his hand,
Was written the name of every saved man.
He spoke not a word as he searched for my name,
When he said "It's not here." My head hung in shame.

The people whose names had been written with love,
He gathered to take to his Father above.
With those who were ready he arose without a sound,
While all the rest were left standing around.

I fell to my knees, but it was too late,
I had waited too long and thus sealed my fate.
I stood and I cried as they arose out of sight,
Oh, if only I had been ready tonight!

In the words of this poem the meaning is clear,
The coming of Jesus is drawing near.
There's only one life and when comes the last call,
We'll find that the Bible was true after all!

Happy Birthday!		Welcome New Associates!	
Nancy Ballinger	12/01	Alvin Anderson	11/23
Alexandra Baptiista	12/19	Buffy Arms	11/09
Deidra Baxter	12/11	Jamie Bloss	11/22
Janie Bybee	12/18	Rick Brady	11/03
Josoph Couch	12/14	Joey Bridges	11/01
Teresa Frost	12/29	Tonya Campbell	11/09
Phillip Glass	12/28	William Cathey	11/16
Melissa Glenn	12/31	Sandee Claborn	11/09
Dora Harrison	12/09	Edward Craig	11/30
Gwendolyn Hines	12/17	Evelio Cunninguam	11/16
Stephanie Hooten	12/20	Kermitt Davis	11/23
Dorothy Hubbell	12/10	Timothy Fitzgerald	11/10
Helen Jackson	12/23	Brian Hamby	11/16
Clarissa Moore	12/23	Janice Haskin	11/16
Gary Roberts	12/25	Gwendolyn Hines	11/08
Horace Roson	12/27	Kayla Holt	11/30
Judith Russell	12/10	Marcella Hudgins	11/23
Sharon Sandles	12/27	Marc Jackson	11/22
Elisabeth Scandrett	12/15	Jennifer Kelley	11/09
Keith Scantlin	12/08	Markecia Knott	11/16
Frances Stiles	12/02	Marsha Lanius	11/02
Kathy Thompson	12/05	Tomyka Lipscomb	11/09
Linda Webster	12/01	Rebecca London	11/16
Carolyn Wright	12/02	Nancy Long	11/06
		Monoca Massey	11/16
		Martha McCall	11/09
		Stephanie McClendon	11/09
		Elissa McNabb	11/16
		Jason Osborne	11/09
		Marianne Paris	11/23
		Jade Piehl	11/30
		Jennifer Pitts	11/09
		Felicia Poulson	11/04
		Teresa Rettig	11/30

	Susan Roberts	11/16
	Jason Roland	11/22
	Peggy Rose	11/09
	Jacqueline Sanchez	11/16
	Troy Smithson	11/23
	Rhonda Thurman	11/09
	Paula Turk	11/09
	James White	11/23

A SAD FAREWELL FROM
MRS. MARTHA.

This will be the hardest letter I have ever written. As of December 31, 1999, I am retiring after 30 years. I am trying to keep it as upbeat as I can, but you can't work as long as I have and not feel like you're losing most of your family at one time.

I have had the last 30 years of my life in retail. Eighteen of them at Wal-Mart and twelve at Big K. There are some of my Big K family still here with me, Betty Hendrix, Bertha Whitaker, and Nelda Baldwin. Some have been with me 18, 17, 16, 10, 11, 12, 9, 7, 5, 4, 3, 2, 1 year(s), and some are so new I haven't had the opportunity to meet.

I just want to say we have laughed, cried and had the best of times and I'll never forget the kindness and prayers that helped me through my husbands illness. I couldn't have made it without you because we are truly a "Wal-Mart Family"

So, keep taking care of our customers and you will be well rewarded, and someday you too can retire and not worry about bills and if you'll have enough money to live on, or if you might be a burden to anyone. I know this may not seem important now, but believe me, my life will be a joy when I retire.

I want to tell you in this letter how much your friendship has meant to me. I love you all and will miss working with you. I won't be able to tell you this in person; I will be too sad.

Enjoy your new store and when you're having a bad day, think of some of the silly things we did or said and maybe it will brighten your day.

Have a Merry Christmas and a Happy New Year,
Martha Lentz
1969 - 1999

Featured Department!

Despite the hectic schedule this time of year I was able to steal a few minutes of time with the manager of this month's featured department, Layaway, a department I am very familiar with! Danielle Jones has been Layaway's department manager since the summer of 1997. Danielle began working at Wal-Mart in August of 1996 as a layaway associate under David Jones (no relation). After David left the following summer, Danielle assumed his position.

Before joining the Wal-Mart family for better pay, Danielle worked at Family Dollar for about three years. Their she performed various duties. Danielle says that some of her favorite things about her job is meeting and working with new people every holiday season and also the customers. The least liked part of her job is during the "off-season" because she likes to stay busy. Danielle says one changes she has seen at Wal-Mart over the past three years is a move toward a more "high tech" approach to retail, which is good since Danielle currently attends Columbia State Community College, where she is pursuing a degree in Computer Programming.

Danielle lives in Mt. Pleasant with her family and her cat Patches, and recently found out she will soon be a aunt. In her spare time Danielle likes to spend time with her friends and her boyfriend, now official fiancé since "the diamond ring", Greg. Danielle would like to express her appreciation to her Layaway staff; Betty, Frances, Jeremy, Kim, Marsha, Matt, Nicole, and "Me", for their hard work during this holiday season.

MONTHLY CONTEST

The Winning Santa Letter!

Jolly Ole Sir. Richard Baud,
    lean your ear this way.
Don't you tell a single soul,
    what I'm going to say.

Martin wants a new sports car,
    Parrish a case of Boost.
Brad needs new roller blades,
    Rob needs a pair too.

Lloyd says a truck is fine,
    any kind at all.
Frank wants a large screen TV,
    and a new VCR.

Martha Lentz doesn't need a
    thing,
    she has more she needs.
Leave her off your list Ole
    Richard,
    she's been bad all year!

Well as for me, a raise is fine,
    gift certificates too.
But cash is mainly on my list,
    see what you can do!

N. Daniel
December 1999

The Walmart Smiley Town News
Volume 1 Issue 9
April 2000

A Note From Richard~

Dear Wal-Mart Associates,

We are really off to a great start for the year 2000! Our sales, along with our profits, are well ahead of last year's. I am convinced that we will reach the $1,000.00 mark for next year's stakeholders bonus! In order to reach this mark we all need to keep focused on our customers. It will take all, working together as a team to accomplish our goals, by doing the following.

- Smile and greet your customers. Show your appreciation to them for shopping with us.
- Keep our store zoned, clean and orderly.
- Keep your Perpetual Inventory correct. This is everyone's job!
- Do your part to keep freight moving out of receiving.

We recently surveyed our associates through the Grass Roots Program. The results are in! The following were found to be the three top issues of concerns with our associates. Along with the issues are the action plans to resolve them. These action plans were formed as a result of our Grass Roots Meetings. I would like to thank everyone of you for your input and willingness to share your ideas.

The first concern of our associates was the hiring of high quality associates. We hope to resolve this issue by actively recruiting career minded students from the local high schools, and also by recruiting students from the local community college, who want to work while attending schools.

The second issue of concern according to the Grass Roots Survey, was management dealing with poor associate performance in a timely and direct manner. We hope to resolve this by involving the immediate supervisor of the associate in the coaching process. We will also assure that our other associates are informed that we are dealing with poor performers.

The last issue of concern was having clean stores. The resolution to this concern involves all associates. You must remember that it is every associates responsibility to pick up trash, hangers, and other litter when you see it. The closing assistant manager will also assign a stockman to clean restrooms and lounges hourly.

In closing, I would like to mention that I am writing this on April 18, 2000, only a few days before Good Friday and Easter. Like most holidays the reason behind them often gets forgotten, our thoughts being on having the extra day off. But, this is such an important event and I hope every one will take a few minutes to reflect on the tremendous sacrifice that was made for you and me 2000 years ago!

Thank you for listening, and may God bless you,
Richard
April 18, 2000

~Happy Birthday~

Victoria Allman	05/29	Jamie Arnold	05/09
Frances Bench	05/27	Joe Brak	05/24
Kathy Cantrell	05/23	Kathrine Dieter	05/20
Frank Fite	05/12	Benjamin Fly	05/06
Carolyn Hight	05/26	Susan Johnson	05/01
Melinda Laroco	05/31	Kathryn Little	05/11
Valerie Logan	05/21	De'Sheria McClain	05/14
Teresa Rettig	05/02	Peggy Rose	05/01
Valerie Sellers	05/11		

~New Associates~

Randall Bradley	03/01	Faylene Brown	03/01
Nathan Carmack	03/16	Melinda Chisler	03/01
Amy Crawford	03/09	Margie Davidson	03/21
Ladona Davis	03/27	Margie Fitzgerald	03/16
Joel Flowers	03/13	Alana Fowler	03/01
Shannon Frost	03/14	Tammy Gallagher	03/16
Linda Glass	03/09	Stanley Glover	03/16
Nicholas Hernandez	03/16	Eric Holford	03/14
David Holland	03/13	Misty Holt	03/16
Shawn Isbell	03/13	Pamela Johnson	03/01
Terry Lopp	03/20	Keith Lowe	03/01
Stephen Lunn	03/01	Kenneth McCafferty	03/18
Michelle Neifert	03/16	Martha Osborne	03/15
Patricia Padgett	03/16	Cassie Ponnwitz	03/09
Terry Ring	03/14	Charles Trupiano	03/14
Muriel Walker	03/01	James Warren	03/01
Cheryl Watts	03/30	Cory Young	03/01

Welcome Our New Associate!

Tammy Gallagher is our new associate for Department 82, Impulse Sells. Tammy helps assure that our checkouts are well stocked with those "can't live without" items, candy being the main one! Tammy, a native of Hohenwald, saw Wal-Mart's "Help Wanted" ad in the local paper. Needing a job to support her two year old son, Austin, Tammy applied and joined our Wal-Mart family in March.

Tammy says her favorite part of the job is meeting the various people and helping them find what they need. Tammy says despite her varying work schedule, she really enjoys working here. There are days when the work never seems too end, and then Tammy says, there are days that are slow. When asked about her future plans, Tammy, who also assist in Department 1, Foods, says along with a big house and a diamond ring, she looks forward to continuing her employment with Wal-Mart. Tammy believes that Wal-Mart is a great company to work for, with good benefits.

With her "spare" time, Tammy, likes to spend it with her son, and an occasional night out at the karaoke bar. Be sure to welcome Tammy to our Wal-Mart family, she is one the most up front and neatest person you could meet.

The Wal-Mart Smiley Town News

April - 2001

Volume 1 Issue 20

A Note From Richard:

Dear Wal-Mart Associates,

In this month's issue, I would like to take the opportunity for some personal reflection.

Over the past three years I have been impressed with how this store's Associates come together to support their fellow Associates. Through sickness, death, or other personal tragedy our Associates are there in times of need. Unfortunately, I now know this support first hand.

In March my oldest brother, Danny, died in his sleep at the age of forty-five. There had been no sign that he was ill, or was having any health problems. This personal tragedy was a shock to me and my entire family. I want to thank all of you who sent cards, letters, expressed sympathy, or let me know that you are praying for my family. Your thoughtfulness is very much appreciated.

From experience I would like to give you some advice of a personal nature. When someone you love dies it is too late to tell them you love them. Don't miss one chance to spend time with your family. Slow down, reflect on your life, and know what is important. Don't be petty or hold grudges. And don't try to win the argument. Life is short, so do yourself a favor and live today like it is your last day on earth.

Most importantly know where you are going to spend eternity! Since Easter is next Sunday I would be remiss if I did not give credit where credit is due. I want to tell you about a friend of mine. His name is Jesus who was sent from Heaven, by God, in the form of a baby born unto a Virgin. He walked the earth thirty-three years spreading the Gospel, telling the world of God's love. He was crucified on a cross and died for our sins.

That is only part of his story. After three days, Jesus rose again, defeating death. He lives today, offering us eternal life if we admit we are sinners and acknowledge that Jesus Christ is God's son who died and rose gain after three days. If you ask Jesus to save you, he promises to do just that.

Again I appreciate all that each and everyone of you do. Not only by doing your job but by being a family to your fellow Associates.

Thank you, and may God bless you.
Richard Baud
April 07, 20001

Business Page Alert!

The **Business Page** will return in the next issue. For now, all associates should be focused on completing the Grass Roots Survey. For assistance contact a member of management or the **Personnel Office**.

WAL-MART SMILEY TOWN NEWS
SEPTEMBER 2001!

VOLUME 1 ISSUE 24

A NOTE FROM RICHARD

Dear Wal-Mart Associates,

This month I will begin this newsletter with a question. Have you ever been the best, the very best, at anything? For example, have your ever been...

- Homecoming King or Queen
- Father Of The Year
- The Star Quarterback
- Club President
- Class Valedictorian
- Chairman Of The Board

Many of us have never been the very best at anything, until Wal-Mart. Do you realize that you, as an Associate of this company, are a part of history. Our Associates are an important part of the world's largest retailer. Wal-Mart is twice the size of both it's nearest competitors combined, and employs more people than any other company in the world.

As part of Wal-Mart's SuperCenter division our store will soon be on the leading edge as the newest, biggest and best part of our company. You may be thinking all that is great, but what does that mean for me? First of all it means job security. Wal-Mart is very profitable, and our company's decisions and goals are long term. This long term commitment is why, when many other companies are failing, Wal-Mart thrives. This allows you, our Associates, to make long term plans with our company. Another important consideration is the opportunities you have with Wal-Mart. Our company has career opportunities in numerous fields such as...

- Buyers
- Computer Specialists
- Information Specialist
- Interrupters
- Pilots
- Real Estate Acquisition

The list continues including, Department Mangers, Assistant Mangers, Store Mangers, and District Managers. You may not know that 74% of our management comes from the hourly Associates ranks.

With our new store there will be many opportunities for you to move up in the company, if you have the abilities and the desire to do so. The bottom line is you are important and can decide the future of our store an our company. Do your best, and be your best every day. If you do that then you won't look back and ask yourself why am I still in this position while everyone else is passing me by. Go ahead, push yourself just a little harder and strive for excellence. Our company is filed with normal ordinary people doing more then they or anyone else ever thought they could do. Lets all do our best and make our current store an example for others to follow and when we move into our new SuperCenter lets show this community what it is to shop in the greatest store they have ever been in.

ANNIVERSARIES

One Year		Two Year	
Constance Gilbreath		Barry Cox	09/08/1999
	09/05/2000	Shannon Ferrara	09/29/1999
Terri McMeen	09/12/2000	Betty Pridy	09/30/1999
Debra Sanders	09/12/2000		
Andrea Sims	09/15/2000		
Norvel Willbanks	09/27/2000		

Three Year		Four Year	
Ryan Blake	09/29/1998	Marye Barnett	09/24/1997
Terri Cox	09/01/1998	Mack Hardison	09/04/1997
Norma Hallmark	09/22/1998	Bernice Young	06/22/1997
Dorothy Hartman	09/22/1998		
Donna Sammons	09/29/1998		

Five Year		Seven Year	
Victoria Allman	09/16/1996	Angela Reynolds	09/05/1994
Vicki Crumley	09/26/1996	Tammy Sells	09/16/1994
Jackie Goodman	09/12/1996		

Eight Year		Eleven Year	
Thelia Thomason	09/21/1993	Debbie Johnson	09/28/1991

Twelve Year		Thirteen Year	
Betty Flewallen	09/13/1989	Helen Jackson	09/01/1988
Dorothy Nichols	09/27/1989		

Fourteen Year		Seventeen Year	
Crawford Crabtree	09/29/1987	Sue Latta	09/28/1986

Seventeen Year		Twenty-Eight Year	
Mora Potts	09/13/1984	Betty Hendrix	09/06/1973

Cathy Armstrong	09/21	Pam Baker	09/30	Pam Beasley	09/05
Nikki Blanchard	09/29	Terry Bowling	09/23	Donna Busby	09/14
Miles Capps	09/17	Trevor Cayce	09/08	Justin Chandler	09/05
Irenella Conger	09/04	Jessica Dirla	09/27	Kendra Frierson	09/03
Constance Gilbreath	09/30	Brenda Gilliam	09/11	Brenda Glenn	09/07
Tonya Hardin	09/23	Gina Hodge	09/09	Patricia Hoffmeyer	09/26
Vivian Johnson	09/13	Lisa Lewsaw	09/16	Walter Long	09/07
Herbert Manning	09/08	Janet Moomaw	09/29	Dorothy Nichols	09/05
Belinda Nolen	09/12	Lillion Page	09/18	Shannon Stonecipher	09/05
Tera Sublet	09/17	Frances Thomason	09/29		

*My apologies to the belated birthday Associates.

WELCOME NEW ASSOCIATES!

Yolanda Brentley	08/30	Rita Briggs	08/16
Debbie Burlison	08/23	Daniel Carter	08/29
Rocky Derryberry	08/08	Larry Estrada	08/08
Melissa Gibson	08/21	Matika Goff	08/15
Leah Gonzales	08/30	Tonya Hardin	08/21
Patricia Hoffmeyer	08/06	Shannon Holliday	08/15
Natasha Hopkins	08/20	Shawn Hopkns	08/14
Jaclyn McMeen	08/15	Martha Miles	08/08
Tion Rollinson	08/16	Dustin Schuesler	08/29
Julie Shores	08/02	Autry Slaughter	08/31

Together We Stand!

On September 11, 2001 the entire world was forever changed. The American people, as a whole, were affected deeply by the tragedies that occurred in New York, Washington, DC and Pennsylvania. Wal-Mart, Sam's Club, and Home Office Associates, are encourage to rise to the occasion and help provide much needed assistance in the massive relief and recovery efforts that are taking place.

The immediate need is for blood donations. All Associates are encourage to work with the local Red Cross or other blood service agencies to assist as need.

The second need is monetary. All Associates are encouraged to give as much as possible to the disaster relief. Collection containers are located throughout our numerous Wal-Mart's and Sam's Clubs. Wal-Mart has committed at least $2 million Dollars to this effort in addition to merchandise, trucks, trailers, and individual efforts across the nation.

Additionally, our walmart.com and samsclub.com websites will have information on our efforts as well as a link to the American Red Cross.

All relief organizations have specifically requested that no merchandise donations be sent, such as food and clothing. The current needs are once again blood and monetary donations.

Any Associates needing counseling, please contact Resources for Living at 1-800-825-3555.

Thank you to all our Associates for all you are doing and continue to do.

A NOTE FROM RICHARD CONTINUED

In a related subject, I would like to recognize a couple of associates who are doing their best each and everyday.

Dala Williams, in HBA, just won the Cabana Cool sales contest. Dala win was for the entire company, and she will be appointed to Wal-Mart's Beauty Advisory Board for one year. Congratulations Dala!

Ryan Blake, from Impulse Merchandising, just received a certificate for achieving a double digit sales increase for the Second Quarter. Congratulations to you also, Ryan

Also congratulations to all of the associates in those departments who helped achieve these results.

Thank you and May God Bless You,
Richard Baud
09/07/2001

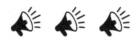

A Note from Richard:

For this month's newsletter article, I felt compelled to write about two topics concerning myself, which is a subject that I feel most uncomfortable about discussing. First on the 15th of December I will be celebrating an anniversary. It was on this date in 1996 that I accepted Jesus Christ as my savior. On that day my Domestics Department Manager gave me a poem to read that God would use to touch my heart and convince me that I needed the Lord. There is a copy of this poem included in this newsletter**. After my acceptance of Christ it was my sole desire in life to make sure that my children would also be saved. I came to find out that by setting an example as their father was a very powerful tool. Once I accepted the Lord, God used my example to open the door for my children to learn about Jesus and within a few months every one of my children accepted the Lord and were saved. Praise God!

Another personal aspect of my life I would like to share is more current and noticeable. In the last five months I have been able to lose over eighty pounds. Many people have asked me how I have lost so much weight. I will touch on that a little later, first I would like to tell you what my motivation was to get busy and lose the weight.

Over the summer my family and I went to Gatlinburg on vacation, returning home on July 4th. On the day of our return I overheard my youngest son say that he had gained thirty pounds in the last few months. That very same day my daughter said that no matter how hard she tried she couldn't get down to the size she wanted to be. At that moment a light went off in my head. I knew that I was responsible for setting a bad example for my children and if I didn't correct it, they would struggle with being overweight for the rest of their lives. So I got busy! I started counting calories and paid closer attention to what and how much I ate. I also began exercising - hard!

---

* *Richard's poem can be found on page 5.*

Like most overweight people I have tried many diets. All ended within a few months, with little loss in weight. This time is different. I am not losing weight for myself. I am motivated to lose weight to set a positive example for my children. For those of you who have asked me how I am losing so much weight, I will tell you the correct question to ask is not how I am losing the weight, but who I am losing it for.

Thank You and May God Bless You
Richard Baud
December 15, 2006

December Anniversaries

One Year
Robert Burks	12/18/2000
Tiffany Miller	12/07/2000
John Skinner	12/13/2005

Three Year
Shannon Mitchell	12/01/2003
Donna Serrett	12/01/2003

Four Year
Charlotte Sorge	12/17/2002

Five Year
Marjorie Morgan	12/03/2001

Six Year
John Brooks	12/18/2000

Seven Year
Wanda Davis	12/08/1999
Kathy Little	12/02/1999

Eight Year
Wilford Mobley	12/15/1998
Marilyn Yant	12/09/1998

Eleven Year
Colleen Slater	12/14/1995

Twelve Year
Audrey Hood	12/01/1994

Twenty-Three Year
Ricky Byrd	12/17/1983

Welcome New

November Associates

Mark Albert	11/14/2006
Myesha Bailey	11/01/2006
Gene Blanchard	11/01/2006
David Boyd	11/14/2006
Danielle Brewer	11/09/2006
Aleshia Buford	11/10/2006
Christyle Bullock	11/29/2006
Rebecca Connelly	11/01/2006
Robert Crigger	11/29/2006
Courtnei Davidson	11/01/2006
Vicki Dunarant	11/07/2006
Brett Emmitt	11/29/2006
Eric Graham	11/29/2006
Tiffany Huey	11/09/2006
Tessa Jennings	11/21/2006
Deborah Love	11/20/2006
Valerie Mayberry	11/10/2006
Jimmy Miller	11/09/2006
Jeff Moore	11/21/2006
Shelia Morton	11/09/2006
Laurie Roberts	11/10/2006
Sulna Santana	11/14/2006
Britini Sharpe	11/17/2006
Tera Shults	11/29/2006
Misty Spicer	11/29/2006
Deah Vandiver	11/06/2006
Leta White	11/14/2006

January Anniversaries

<u>Three Year</u>
Stephanie Clingerman   01/06/2004
Walter Mears, Jr.   01/19/2004
Brenda Paschall   01/29/2004

<u>Five Year</u>
"Travis" Bonney   01/28/2002
Betty Ferguson   01/30/2002
Rachel Larkin   01/28/2002
Sharon Sewell   01/28/2002

<u>Thirteen Year</u>
Mary Ingram   01/24/1994

<u>Twenty-Five Year</u>
Sheree Brady   01/18/1982

Welcome New

January Associates!

Vikki Bolton   12/12/2006
Cynthia Hutcherson   12/15/2006
Amanda Potts   12/07/2006
Lisa Privette   12/07/2006
Susan Slaughter   12/12/2006
Christopher Whitwell   12/07/2006

Just For Fun!

The Three Stages of Life (Christmas Style)

1. You believe in Santa Claus
2. You don't believe in Santa Claus
3. You are Santa Claus

RECIPE FOR CHRISTMAS JOY

Ingredients:

1/2 cup Hugs
4 tsp Kisses
2 cups Smiles
4 cups Love
1 cup Special Holiday Cheer
1/2 cup Peace on Earth
3 tsp Christmas Spirit
2 cups Goodwill Toward Man
1 Sprig of Mistletoe
1 Med.-size bag of Christmas Snowflakes

Mix Hugs, Kisses, Smiles and Love until consistent. Blend in Holiday Cheer, Peace on Earth, Christmas Spirit and the Good Will toward Men. Use the mixture to fill a large, warm heart, where it can be stored for a lifetime. (It never goes bad!) Serve as desired under Mistletoe, sprinkled liberally with Christmas Snowflakes. It is especially good when accompanied by Christmas Carols and family get-togethers.

Serve to one and all.

~

When you stop believing in Santa Claus is when you start getting clothes for Christmas.

BLUE CHRISTMAS

This information was obtained on the WIRE.

There is a holiday song that includes the verse *"It's the most wonderful time of the year."* While this is true for most of us this Christmas Season, for many people in the midst of depression this time of the year brings about further complications.

Depression might be the temporary sadness that follows a loss or it might be a more disruptive illness that interferes with the ability to enjoy work and family life. Often the depressed person is overwhelmed by feelings of hopelessness and inaction, which make it difficult for the person to reach out to others. But depression can be treated with combinations of support, medical intervention and self-help. The most important thing is for the person to reach out for help.

One such way to obtain supportive help is through counseling. We as Wal-Mart Associates are fortunate that we are able to obtain free professional counseling and consultation as one of the benefits of our employment. These telephone services are provided by Resources For Living (RFL) for all full-time and part-time Wal-Mart Associates and their immediate family members. Each of the phone counselors have a master's degree in a counseling field such as marriage and family therapy, clinical psychology, counseling psychology, or social work. This educational requirement ensures that RFL counselors maintain very high professional standards in the industry.

One of the RFL counselors core belief is the capability of people. They use their professional skills and experience to provide support and help with issues that concern you. They work with you to explore a variety of options, solutions, or resources that may be most helpful. They work to empower you to make the best decisions possible.

Resources For Living maintains the highest standards of confidentiality within legal and ethical guidelines. RFL does not release the identity of a caller or any personally identifying information to leaders in field locations or the home office. Resources For Living counselors may only break confidentiality when it is necessary to protect someone who is at risk of harm.

Almost everyone who experiences feelings of depression recovers and feels good again. It's a step-by-step process but the first small step leads to the next one and, with help, you'll be able to cope with life again.

Resources For Living
1-800-825-3555
www.rfl.com

Peace on
Earth

TWAS THE NIGHT BEFORE
JESUS CAME

Twas the night before Jesus came and all through the house,
Not a creature was praying, not one in the house.
Their Bibles were lain on the shelf without care,
In hopes that Jesus would not come there.

The children were dressing to crawl into bed,
Not once ever kneeling or bowing a head.
And Mom in the rocker with Baby on her lap,
Was watching the Late Show while I took a nap.

When out of the East there arose such a clatter,
I sprang to my feet to see what was the matter.
Away to the window I flew like a flash!
Tore open the shutters and threw up the sash!

When what to my wondering eyes should appear,
But angels proclaiming that Jesus was here!
With a light like the sun sending forth a bright ray,
I knew in a moment this must be the day.

The light of his face made me cover my heard,
It was Jesus returning just like he said.
And though I possessed worldly wisdom and wealth,
I cried when I saw him in spite of myself.

In The Book of Life which he held in his hand,
Was written the name of every saved man.
He spoke not a word as he searched for my name,
When he said "It's not here." My head hung in shame.

The people whose names had been written with love,
He gathered to take to his Father above.
With those who were ready he arose without a sound,
While all the rest were left standing around.

I fell to my knees, but it was too late,
I had waited too long and thus sealed my fate.
I stood and I cried as they arose out of sight,
Oh, if only I had been ready tonight!

In the words of this poem the meaning is clear,
The coming of Jesus is drawing near.
There's only one life and when comes the last call,
We'll find that the Bible was true after all!

Chapter 5 Walmart

On 2-19-2006 I gave my testimony to my Church, this Testimony included telling about my Daughter Katherine Baud,

Here is what I said about her.

On Katie's first week of high school, her Freshmen year she was in science class and got into a discussion about God and how to be Saved And Katie lead a fellow student to the Lord in the middle of science class.

Then in the last Revival at our Church Katie was troubled about a little neighbor girl that she had befriended several years ago when the girl was 5 or 6, the Preacher was preaching about Hell and not letting your family or friends go there, Katie had told the little girl about Hell and how to be Saved years ago, but after that the girl's parents stopped letting her play with Katie and she had lost track of her. In that Revival meeting Katie told me and Ramona that she had to go and talk to that girl now!! of course we first thought of how late it was and how it might appear (knocking on someone's door at 9 pm on a Wednesday night) But Katie would have none of it she was determined to go and talk to her little friend and Save her from Hell. So after Revival I took Katie to the house the girl had lived in. We expected to see the girl and her parents come to the door, instead this 50+ year old man with a New Jersey accent came to the door, Katie asked the man where the little girl was and the man said that the family had moved 6 months ago and that he now lived there. I thought well that is it let's go home, but Katie had no intention of giving up she told the man about Revival and that she had been told to go to this house tonight because someone there needed the Lord and she didn't want anyone to go to Hell.

He along with myself were both amazed. He said (young lady you have got the wrong house) and Katie said (if you die today will you go to Heaven or Hell? are you Saved?) he said I am probably not Saved like you think Saved means but I have been to a Church before, Katie continued and thru her own tears told him that Jesus loved him and didn't want him to go to Hell she told him the plan of Salvation, he stood there and listened with great interest in what she said he then turned Katie away. She invited him to Revival and told him that she would pray for him.

I do not know if that man has been Saved but I know that Katie did her part in sharing Jesus. And God's word will eventually bear fruit.

I am 44 years old and that was the bravest thing that I have ever seen, I am very proud of Katie she gives us big brave adults an example of being bold for God.

Thank you and may God bless you.

2-19-2006

The reason that I included the story of my brave 16 year old daughter in this Walmart chapter is that I would also be challenged to live out my Faith later in 2006.

I will not go into detail about it, but Walmart had been involved in a major controversy concerning our company supporting a national gay and lesbian group.

The next story takes place at Walmart's fall holiday meeting with every store manager in the company attending including me.

On the morning of 9-10-2006, I went to Walmart's Chapel service, during this service I talked to God and asked him to lead me and if it was his will for me to take a stand for him at Walmart, I asked him to put the CEO of Walmart Lee Scott in my path so that I could speak to him. I really wanted not to see Lee Scott, it would have been easier for me just to mail the letter I had prepared for him and the Chairman of the Board of Walmart Rob Walton, after I had returned home.

On Sunday 9-10-2006 at 2pm I nearly walked into the CEO of Walmart Lee Scott, I took one look at him and thought to myself oh no!! That instant I knew that God had put Lee Scott in my path so I said to myself hello Richard this is it, you either stand up for what you believe or chicken out and regret it the rest of your life. As I approached Lee, the 4 or 5 people that were around him left and it was just him and me so I took a deep breath and went up to Lee, I handed him the envelope that contained the letter that I had earlier prepared for him. He took the envelope and looked at me, I said Lee this is a letter that I wrote you, please read it when you can, then I got braver and I said, what this is about is Walmart supporting the National gay and lesbian group, Lee said Walmart is not supporting that group, I said there has been a press release from the group saying that Walmart is a member and there has been newspaper articles saying the same thing. Lee said what happened is that a low level home office associate who is gay joined the national gay and lesbian group by himself, not on behalf of Walmart. Then the national gay and lesbian group immediately sent out a press release stating that Walmart is a member of and supports their group, he said this is not true he also said we will not pay for same sex partner health insurance benefits.

I then said that if that is the case then Walmart needs to correct the record and let the public know that we do not support that group Lee said that Walmart had decided not to say anything, they preferred just to let the issue die. I told Lee that I didn't want to tell him how to do his job but this is a big deal, that it had upset Christians that Walmart would support such a group and that local preachers were passing out copies of the national gay and lesbian group's press release and were preaching against shopping at Walmart. In addition to that, I have had lots of people calling me and telling me in person that they were concerned about Walmart supporting this group and that they would stop shopping at Walmart. Lee said that Walmart was in the middle of a lot of issues like plan b abortion pill and immigration and that Walmart could not win either way, he said that the whole Walmart supporting the gay and lesbian group issue would blow over in a couple of weeks. I told Lee that I personally was concerned about this and that I would suggest that he set the record straight. Lee said that he didn't want to appear that we were anti gay or against any group, I told Lee that Jesus said that we should love everyone. I added that even though we should love everyone, we should not support something that God is against, Lee said I guess God will sort it out after we die. Lee left and went his way.

I have attached a copy of the letter that I handed Lee Scott, I also mailed both Lee Scott and Rob Walton a copy of this letter.

Dear Mr. Rob Walton and Mr. Lee Scott,

My name is Richard Baud and I am currently the Store Manager of Columbia Tennessee Wal-Mart.

I am writing to you because of the announcement by Wal-Mart that our company has recently made a $25,000 contribution to the NGLCC (National Gay & Lesbian Chamber of Commerce) and Wal-Mart has now developed a partnership with this group.

The reason that I chose to write to both of you is simply that you have the power to either make or seriously influence decisions that affect every associate and every member of management that works for our company.

I started my career with Wal-Mart at age 19 on 12-30-80 and I have been a loyal Wal-Mart employee over these many years working hard along with my co-workers to help build our company. Shortly after I began with Wal-Mart I was assigned to the Taylorville, IL store as Assistant Manager. There in early 1982 I had my first in person meeting with our founder Sam Walton. As Sam Walton normally did he met with our management team after he toured our store. It was at that meeting in our snack bar that Sam asked me which company I had worked for prior to Wal-Mart and why I had left them. During our discussion I told him that my previous company treated people badly and their executives took kickbacks from vendors and at corporate functions hard liquor was served. Then Sam Walton told me that I had made a good choice at coming to Wal-Mart. Sam said that he and his family believed in the golden rule – Do unto others as you would have them do unto you. Sam said that Wal-Mart would always use the Good Book – The Bible, as its guide in its dealings.

I have always been proud of our company taking a stand, for example when Wal-Mart edited music and took out materials that were unfit to be sold in a Wal-Mart store.

I am not sure how Wal-Mart made the decision to publicly and proudly proclaim its partnership with this organization, but I do know that this puts Wal-Mart on the wrong side of the Bible and what God finds acceptable.

You two gentlemen have a huge responsibility in leading a giant like Wal-Mart; millions of people, Wal-Mart associates, vendors, and customers depend on Wal-Mart and Wal-Mart due to its size and success is a leader. Many companies will follow Wal-Mart's lead and go down the same path.

I respectfully am asking for you two leaders to stand up for what is morally right and reverse this decision and return Wal-Mart back to where our founder Sam Walton left it A moral leader in our nation where our associates can be proud to work and our customers can be proud to shop.

I realize that I am only one person and that my voice is weak but I pray that you both will take my request into consideration. I believe that Wal-Mart has been richly blessed by God over the years and by turning away from God Wal-Mart will no longer enjoy these blessings.

Thank you for reading and considering my request,

May God Bless You,

Richard Baud
9-8-06

This is a picture that I sent (along with my letter) to Lee Scott and Rob Walton, the picture is of me and Sam Walton that was taken in 1981 when Sam Walton visited the Walmart store in Taylorville Illinois.

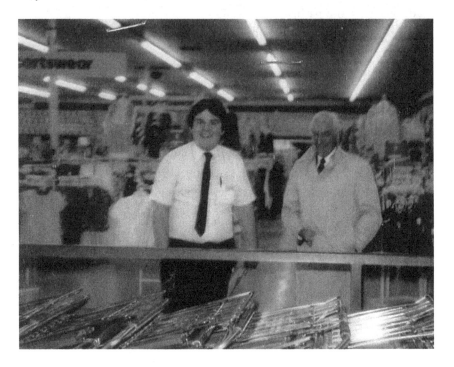

After I spoke to Lee Scott I knew that I had done my part and as my Daughter had showed me back 7 months earlier that, what God wants us to do is our part.

As time moved on my family progressed and one by one each of our four children left home to start their own families, as this happened I found myself growing even closer to my Walmart family.

At Walmart even though some Associates leave every year, others stay and new Associates are hired so I had an awesome Walmart family to focus on as I "reluctantly" at home became an Empty Nester.

I would lean on my Walmart family as my kids left home one at a time, as my oldest brother died and as my Mother died, it is good to have such a big family.

I will skip ahead to the year 2020, this is the year that Covid-19 hit the world including our store. Since the Pandemic experience was the first one in over 100 years Walmart like every other Company in the World had to figure stuff out in real time.

The entire Nation was in pure panic mode as people around the Country started to die of Covid-19, Walmart would start having our Associates wear masks asking everyone to social distance and asking our customers to wear masks and limit the operating hours for the store.

At the store level our Associates and management staff were faced with issue after issue with. Our corporation constantly changing direction

1. on how many customers could be in the store at one time.
2. on how to keep our customers spaced out 6 foot apart.
3. on forcing our customers to wear masks.
4. on weather to limit the quantities that customers could buy of certain products like toilet paper paper towels cleaning and sanitizing supplies meat e.t.c.
5. on the store hours of operation.

Almost always the company direction would be complicated and very hard to execute at the store level, At the same time our customers were split between those who were scared to death and wanted everything possible to be done to limit the spread of Covid-19 and those who were not worried about the possibility of getting or spreading the disease so our team of Associates and management had to navigate between these factions while working even harder to keep the store stocked, clean and taking care of our customers.

During these very trying times our store came thru big time, as many Associates would call out due to having Covid-19 or calling out because they were afraid that they might get Covid-19 if they were around so many customers, and as our company required lots of Associates to be involved in checking Associates temperatures as they arrived for work and monitoring customer compliance with Covid-19 rules and constant cleaning. This left fewer Associates to actually run the store but those who were left working were true heroes.

Even though many were scared themselves of getting Covid-19 they did what they needed to, to keep the store stocked and clean and our customers taken care of dealing with lots of product shortages and irate customers and ever changing Covid-19 rules.

During the Covid-19 crisis in August of 2020, I started to have some health issues, I started having problems including with my right knee, and with my right shoulder I had to put more effort into doing what I normally did with ease but I kept going, doing the best job possible with my new physical limitations and a wild Covid-19 environment, I had decided that I would retire from Walmart on 2-1-2021, I wanted to spend more time with my grandchildren the oldest of my grandchildren would be turning 13 in April of 2021, as it turns out I would not be able to retire.

From the day that I was Saved on 12-15-1996, I knew that I was not alone and could count on God. I started my day on 11-18-2020 like normal I said my prayers including asking God to protect me at work, I have the confidence that if God wants me to do something then he will make it possible for me to do it, and once he does not want me to do something God will nudge me to where he wants me to go. As I have previously written when we went from Manassas Virginia to Columbia Tennessee in 1998, God had shut many doors and nudged us out of Virginia only to put us in a better position in Tennessee.

So 11-18-2020 was like many days in Covid-19 Walmart, full of lots of challenges including 23 Associates on Covid-19 leave of absence in addition to the normal Associate call outs.

As the day progressed our Market manager arrived and was not happy with the condition of the store, the store like all Walmarts has good days and bad days where things do not come together well this was one of the those days.

Long story short the Market manager told me to go home and that he would contact the Regional Vice President and ask for his permission to terminate my employment with Walmart, he said that he would contact me later that day with the verdict.

I knew that this was the end, the Market manager had found the store in a condition that he could justify terminating me I also knew that the Regional Vice President would go along with the termination because I had burned my bridges with him over my argument about the decision on the personnel manager position.

So I went home and asked God to allow me to represent him well as I was being terminated I asked God to allow me to leave my Walmart career with an attitude of gratitude for what Walmart had allowed me to do in life. Later that day the market manager called and informed me that I would be terminated and he asked me to come back to the store the next day to fill out the needed paperwork.

So on 11-19-20 I returned to the Walmart store that I managed for 22 years and was officially terminated ending a career that started on 12-30-1980.

At my final meeting with the market manager I tried to go out with the proper respect including showing restraint when the market manager told me that Walmart had passed me by and not to worry because the same thing happens to everyone eventually, so I left the store, my only regret was that I could not properly express to my Walmart Associates how much that I appreciated them. These folks had become my family and I lost them all in one day. So I will express my appreciation now to all of the wonderful Associates and amazing management team from my Walmart store 0192, you have been a big part of my life for 22 years and I thank you for all the support and Love that you have given me all these years. I wish everyone the very best, I hope that God will bless each and everyone of you.

I look forward to seeing everyone around our community in the months and years to come as for me I will do what I planned on doing when I was to retire on 2-1-2021, I will spend as much time as I can with my kids and my grandchildren and I will look to God as to what happens next in my life.

I will end this Walmart chapter with some general thoughts about Walmart

First, the Associates run the store, management at all levels come and go.

Second, Walmart Associates work very hard and care about their jobs.

Third, at Walmart the Associates form a type of family, they look out for each other and are there when someone has a life changing problem, many times Associates raise money to help someone down on their luck.

Fourth, you can usually tell if a new Associate will be successful by how they were raised, if they had a loving family and a good support system they would usually make a good productive Associate if not then they have a very small chance of being a long term associate. Many times a new Associate will have a car break down or a baby sitter problem or an ex-spouse issue that prevents them from coming to work and after a while they leave the company or are terminated from their position. If that associate would have had a family support system they would have been able to overcome those issues.

Fifth, many times an irate customer takes their frustrations out on the closest associate even cussing the Associate or threatening violence on the associate, no one has the right to treat an employee of Walmart or any other retailers or any other service type company with disrespect remember that person could be your Son or Daughter and they are just trying to do their job.

Sixth, when Walmart had an associate trampled to death in New York on Black Friday Walmart learned the wrong lesson from the experience, they should have decided that the entire concept was bad and puts customers and Walmart associates in danger and should be canceled and replaced with smaller more focused sales spread out over the entire Christmas season to limit the chaos due to so many people coming into a store in such a short time frame, instead they decided to put tons of rules and procedures in place to control the crowds, making a tough job turn into a nightmare try to manage Black Friday.

Seventh, Walmart started going down a deceitful path when they decided to change the district manager position making it into a market manager position, changing job descriptions and making the district managers apply for this renamed position, using this process to terminate many long term district managers and replacing them with younger more technologically sound people under the new position of market manager.

This process would continue to be used to downsize positions in the company including the co-manager position the assistant manager position and the personnel managers position, Walmart is transitioning its workforce which is needed but using this process is not a fair way of doing it.

CHAPTER 6

MOM

This Chapter is dedicated to my Mom, my mom was an imperfect Woman who made lots of mistakes in her life but she was very determined and set an example for me in how to never give up and keep moving forward regardless of how many obstacles that are thrown in your way. My Mom was born on 9-28-1937 to a large family that included her Father who was a Preacher. My mom's family was poor like most people during those Depression era years. My mom told me many times how she hated to fish because she and her Siblings had to fish (while she was a child) to help feed the family, since my mom was a child during World War 2 she had lots of memories of those times including seeing Adolf Hitler as a real life Monster, mom said that she would see posters and even cartoons depicting Hitler this way, mom said that she had many nightmares about Hitler.

My mom's Father died in a terrible accident involving his car running into a train while she was still a young child.

At the age of 17 my mom got pregnant and left home marrying her first husband Bill Ruffner.

Mom had four children with her first husband, they later divorced, then my mom married my Father (her second husband) Paul Baud, mom had 3 children with her second husband, after the second Child my parents divorced, it was only after that divorce that my mom found out that she was pregnant with a third child from her second husband. My mom gave that child up for adoption to one of her Brothers, this man and his wife were in a good position in life where they could easily afford to raise a child.

My mom met and later married James Grieves, this man was my

step father as I was growing up, mom and her third husband had two children, her third husband died of Cancer on 2-18-1980.

As I was growing up I could always count on my mom, mom worked hard and did whatever she had to do to raise me and my seven Brothers and Sisters (as I was growing up I was not told about the Brother that was Adopted out) it was on my 18th Birthday that mom informed me about the existence of this Brother.

Over the years mom who was very busy raising me and my seven Siblings, worked different jobs outside of the home to help make ends meet including a factory in Oblong Illinois named Standard Grigsby, mom also worked as a waitress and finally worked at the Candy Factory in Robinson Illinois, mom worked there until she retired at the age of 70.

My mom loved Country Music I remember her playing record albums of some of the greats in her day including.

Conway Twitty
George Jones
Patsy Cline
Loretta Lynn
Johnny Cash

My mom was definitely the one in charge in the family she was tough, what she said she meant and she did not expect to have to tell you twice to do something.one of her favorite things to say was "I brought you into this World and I can take you out of it"

I can only remember seeing my mom cry twice the first time was after our house burnt to the ground we had to move to a much smaller house, one day it got to her, everyone of us kids seemed to have an issue as mom was trying to get us ready to go to school, mom finally said forget it you are all staying home from school today, as the tears went down her face.

The second time that I seen my mom cry was when she found out that her mother had died, mom quickly ran into the bathroom as tears ran down her face, other then those two times I never seen my mom cry, she was a very strong Woman.

Mom came to my rescue when I was in the sixth grade, I had skipped school and forged my mom's signature on a note to excuse me from being absent from school.

My handwriting has never been good and the school figured out that the note was fake, the school called my mom to get her approval to spank me, my mom told the principal that if anyone was going to spank me that it would be her, it blew up into a big thing I ended up being suspended from school for three days

So I skipped school and my punishment was missing three more days of school, I loved it!, and my mom was so mad at the school that she never really punished me for skipping school and forging her signature.

I give my Mom all the credit for any success in life that I have had, she set a great example of how to work hard and be focused on the task at hand. When I was promoted to management at Pamida, my Mom and her sister my Aunt Louellen were shopping at Pamida and my mom was bragging to Aunt Louellen about how proud she was of me becoming a member of management at the age of 18 as they turned a corner there I was, on my hands and knees scraping up gum from the floor, mom and Aunt Louellen laughed and laughed at the situation, not a glamorous job but I did whatever I needed to do to be successful at my job.my Mom was a stubborn person, another trait that she passed down to me.my Mom had a bad experience when she first tried to learn how to drive a vehicle, this included several of her children being tossed around in her car, mom did not drive again until she was 55 years old, her last grown child was leaving home and Mom had to learn to drive or be stuck at home, so she learned how to drive. Mom never liked to back up and one time at a gas station mom pulled in and pumped her gas and intended to continue driving forward when another lady got in my moms path and expected my mom to back up and let her continue driving forward a standoff started between mom and the other lady, mom never backed up out waiting the other lady, once the lady left then mom continued pulling forward and left the gas station..

When mom was diagnosed with Cancer my mom was determined to beat it and fought hard to overcome it, during this time her insurance paid for mom to have an (at home) Physical Therapist, mom did not like to take orders from anyone and this included her physical therapist, mom would argue constantly with her physical therapist and eventually the physical therapist would quit or mom would fire them.

Eventually it would be a real struggle for mom to continue living at home by herself she would do things like leaving the stove on and not using her walker to move around her house, causing many dangerous falls.so on 7-2-2011 mom had to go to a nursing home (the same one that her mother had stayed in prior to her death) mom had always said that she would never go to a nursing home, so the day that she was forced to go to that nursing home mom was terribly upset showing her anger at employees of the nursing home, family members and everyone else that was in the vicinity. Mom eventually settled in and made the best out of it but was not at all pleased that she was there. The last time I talked to mom was on a Wednesday night and mom told me that she had got in trouble, apparently you are supposed to eat all of the food on your plate and mom did not like peas so she moved her peas off of her plate onto another woman's plate, and this other lady narked out my mom.

My mother did not have it easy in life and made some difficult decisions.

1. when she was 17 years old she got pregnant and chose to keep the baby and got married.
2. when I was two years old my mother divorced my father who was a drunk, at that time she had 6 children, then she found out that she was pregnant with child # 7 my mom gave that child up for adoption providing a family that could not have any children an awesome blessing, mom could have made another very bad choice and Aborted her baby.

As I was growing up my family rarely went to Church and there was no talk about God in our household. I was saved on 12-15-1996 since that day I started to reach out to my extended family witnessing to them thru letters and when possible in person, I had them in my prayers daily asking God to intervene and Save their Souls, really my efforts seemed to fall on deaf ears including with my mom.my mom was a tough customer even making the comment that I was becoming one of those religious fanatics. Then my mom got sick and our Church, The Northside Baptist Church in Columbia Tennessee started praying for her, in addition to praying for mom my Church had members that would send my mom get well letters and greeting cards, one member of my Church family (Lois Lindsey) sent my mom tons of cards and letters and they meant so much to my mom, mom would tell me this every time I would call her. For the entire 6 years from the day mom was diagnosed with Cancer, Northside Baptist Church continued to pray for my mom and to send those awesome cards and letters to her.

Very gradually my mom began to listen to what I had to say about Jesus and mom was touched so much by the kind words from Lois Lindsey, Lois was able to make a connection with mom and thru those cards and letters was able to share Jesus with my mom, I once thought that it was sad that my mom had to get sick in order to warm up to the Gospel but now I know it took that to wake her up.

As my mom got sicker she realized that her death was coming and she finally realized that she needed Jesus. I had several discussions with my mom about her salvation and I thought that she had been Saved, but I was not sure. So I prayed to God that he would give me one more chance to be sure that mom was saved.

I asked God to allow me some time alone with her and that she would be alert and receptive to God's plan of Salvation, I went to see my mom in the hospital on Friday night 7-15-2011 when I got there my mom was alert and alone, we had a nice talk and she brought up the fact that she probably was not going to get better and did not think that she would live much longer, mom said that she was ready to be with God.

I asked her if she was sure about her Salvation, she was not sure, so I asked her if I could share God's plan of Salvation with her, mom asked me to.

I used the (Roman Road) and shared God's plan of Salvation with her including

Romans 3:23
Romans 5:8
Romans 6:23
Romans 10:9, 10
Romans 10:13

Next is a copy of the Roman Road.

THE ROMAN ROAD

Jesus prepared for us a simple plan of salvation. Presented in the Book of Romans of the Holy Bible, this outline will show you step by step how to be saved.

ROMANS 3:23
"For all have sinned, and come short of the glory of God." — ALL have sinned —

ROMANS 5:8
"But God commendeth his love toward us, in that, while we were yet sinners, Christ died for us" — ALL are loved —

ROMANS 6:23
"For the wages of sin is death, but the gift of God is eternal life through Jesus Christ our Lord." — The PAYMENT for sin is death, separation from God forever But salvation is a GIFT from God, not earned by going to church, baptism, good works, etc. —

ROMANS 10:9, 10
"That if thou shalt confess with thy mouth the Lord Jesus, and shalt believe in thine heart that God hath raised him from the dead, THOU SHALT BE SAVED." "For with the heart man believeth unto righteousness; and with the mouth confession is made unto salvation." — Just BELIEVE and RECEIVE —

ROMANS 10:13
*For WHOSOEVER shall can upon the name of the Lord SHALL BE SAVED."

**AFTER FOLLOWING THE PLAN OF
SALVATION LEAD THEM IN THIS PRAYER**

Dear Lord Jesus, I'm a Sinner — I'm Lost. I Need to be Saved. I Want to be Saved. If You Will Save Me, I'll Give You My Life. Thank You Jesus for Saving Me.

**— After praying this prayer, go over the scriptures
on the other side of this card —**

My mom accepted the Lord as her Savior at 1030 pm that night 7-15-2011 Praise the Lord!

After my mom passed away on Sunday 7-24-2011, I asked God to give me peace about my mother, then on my way home from Illinois back to Columbia Tennessee I turned the car radio on to a Gospel station, the very first words that I heard from that song was (she is in a better place)

God is good!

My mother is in Heaven and I'm not worried about her anymore but I am concerned about my brothers and sisters who are not Saved.

I spoke to the preacher who was to preach my mom's Funeral the day before my mom's Funeral, he had worked with my mom for 10 years at the local Hershey candy factory before my mom had retired.

I asked him if he had ever asked my mom about her Salvation, he had not. I told him about her Salvation experience and I asked him to use the Funeral to witness to members of my family who might be more receptive to the message if they knew that my mom had accepted the Lord, he was a little hesitant but said that he would.

God heard my prayers and the prayers from my Church family, because at my mother's Funeral that (hesitant Preacher) preached a Sermon.

During the Sermon he said that he had been up since 3 am wrestling with what to say, he could not rest!!

During the sermon he was very direct

1. he said that my mom (who loved to gamble) had gambled with her eternal life to the very last minute.
2. he said that if they ever wanted to see mom again that they would need to follow mom's example and accept the Lord as their Personal Savior, he then shared God's plan of Salvation.
3. he spoke of Jesus and how God had sent him to die for our sins.
4. I could see people around the room listening carefully

I believe that Sermon will lead to many great things for my family over the years.

I would ask all that read this book to please pray for my Siblings that they all will accept the Lord as their Savior and be Saved.

On 9-4-2011 I spoke to my Church family at Northside Baptist Church, I thanked the Church members for all of their prayers cards and letters over the past 6 years and I told them about my mom accepting the Lord and about all that had went on at her Funeral, after I was done sharing that Testimony, Betty Smith who was a Sunday School teacher for four and five year olds while I was Sunday School Director came over to me and told me that on the night my mom was saved 7-15-2011, she Betty Smith woke up from a dream where she was told to pray for my mom, so she prayed for my moms Salvation at the very time that mom accepted the Lord.

Praise God

CHAPTER 7

NORTHSIDE
BAPTIST CHURCH

This chapter is about a Church that has been an important part of my life since our family moved to Columbia in 1998.

I know that one reason God moved my family to Columbia is Northside Baptist Church, as I have previously mentioned in other chapters of this book, after visiting basically every Baptist Church in town we choose Northside Baptist Church because of one line that then Pastor John Rushing repeatedly said "we need to keep the main thing the main thing" meaning that the Church should concentrate on sharing Jesus with others and by doing so see people Saved by the blood of Jesus. This same phrase and devotion to seeing people Saved was also the focus of our Church in Virginia (Battlefield Baptist Church), so Northside Baptist Church was a natural fit for our family and as it turned out, many blessings would come to our family thru Northside Baptist Church, I want to share a few of those blessings now.

First, on 11-7-1999 during a Revival service our daughter Katie accepted Jesus as her personal Savior. Second, on 9-28-2003 my youngest son Samuel asked one of his fellow Church youth group members (Lauren Cole) to go out with him, this lead to Samuel and Lauren getting married on 6-16-2007 and then on 5-20-20 their Son, my sixth grandchild Albert was born.

Third, thanks to the many cards and letters and prayers for my mom's Salvation from Northside Baptist Church to my mom over several years, my mom would accept Jesus as her personal Savior on 7-15-2011.

I also was able to grow in my journey as a Christian by accepting the responsibility of becoming the Sunday School Director at Northside starting in 1998 and continuing for ten years, I learned that to be a good Sunday School Teacher you have to have the goal to teach Jesus and see people Saved thru Sunday School. A good Sunday School Teacher will do some very important things including.

1. reaching out to non Christians, invite them to Sunday School class and teach them about Jesus.
2. they must care about the Souls of their Sunday school class members.
3. they will visit the sick in the hospital or in their homes.
4. they will go to funerals of those who die in order to help comfort family members.
5. they will call or send cards to Sunday school members who miss a Sunday school class.

As the years went by I was able to share my testimony with the congregation of Northside Baptist Church, next I am attaching a copy of those testimonies.

MY TESTIMONY GIVEN AT NORTHSIDE BAPTIST CHURCH ON 2 - 17 - 2002

Good morning, in order to give my Testimony I need to begin at the beginning of my life and let you know where I came from, First of all I was born in a small town in Illinois, I was one of 8 kids, my mother was married 3 times, as we were growing up our family was very poor. My grandfather on my mother's side was killed in a car/train accident before I was born, and my grandfather on my father's side was killed in a refinery accident when I was 2 years old, I. Mentioned earlier that my mother had been married 3 times, her second husband was my father, my parents were divorced when I was 3 years old, my father had a serious drinking problem, after my parents divorced even though my father lived within 10 miles from me, to this date I have only seen him 7 or 8 times my entire life, most of my memories of my family were after my mother married her third husband who was 20 years older then her (he died of cancer when I was 18 years old) I have 2 older sisters who both dropped out of high school and were married after becoming pregnant. My 2 older brothers were both always in trouble, in and out of jail from the time they were 16 years old. I know now that God had to be looking out for me or I would of never had a chance in life. Our family never discussed God and went to Church only 2 or 3 times my entire childhood. I still remember a couple of times my stepfather slammed the door on visiting Pastors, well I made it through those years and thru Walmart I was able to do ok in life, but I still did not know God, once I met Ramona I began to realize that her family was very different than mine, her family all went to Church and they knew the Lord. After we were married we went to Church occasionally and I began to learn a little about religion and Church life, over the years as we moved with Walmart we would go to Church occasionally, only for Worship service, then one fall day in 1995 our family was out for a ride in the country when we passed by a Church, my youngest son looked up at the Church and said Daddy what does that T stand for? God told me that very minute that I needed to get and keep my family in Church, so we went to the Church he had pointed to and started going every week, I had a new commitment to learn for myself what that T stood for, we had a very good Preacher who told it like it is, each week I felt the Lord telling me to accept him as my Savior, but I was stubborn and resisted, then in December of 1996 one of my department managers at Walmart gave me this poem (Read it now) I was immediately convicted and made the decision to accept the Lord, that Sunday 12-15-1996 I walked down the aisle and accepted Jesus as my Savior, the Bible says that Jesus will save whosoever asks him to, I beg of you, if you do not know Jesus, accept him today before it is everlasting too late.

Thank you and may God bless you.

TWAS THE NIGHT BEFORE
JESUS CAME

Twas the night before Jesus came and all through the house,
Not a creature was praying, not one in the house.
Their Bibles were lain on the shelf without care,
In hopes that Jesus would not come there.

The children were dressing to crawl into bed,
Not once ever kneeling or bowing a head.
And Mom in the rocker with Baby on her lap,
Was watching the Late Show while I took a nap.

When out of the East there arose such a clatter,
I sprang to my feet to see what was the matter.
Away to the window I flew like a flash!
Tore open the shutters and threw up the sash!

When what to my wondering eyes should appear,
But angels proclaiming that Jesus was here!
With a light like the sun sending forth a bright ray,
I knew in a moment this must be the day.

The light of his face made me cover my heard,
It was Jesus returning just like he said.
And though I possessed worldly wisdom and wealth,
I cried when I saw him in spite of myself.

In The Book of Life which he held in his hand,
Was written the name of every saved man.
He spoke not a word as he searched for my name,
When he said "It's not here." My head hung in shame.

The people whose names had been written with love,
He gathered to take to his Father above.
With those who were ready he arose without a sound,
While all the rest were left standing around.

I fell to my knees, but it was too late,
I had waited too long and thus sealed my fate.
I stood and I cried as they arose out of sight,
Oh, if only I had been ready tonight!

In the words of this poem the meaning is clear,
The coming of Jesus is drawing near.
There's only one life and when comes the last call,
We'll find that the Bible was true after all!

MY TESTIMONY GIVEN AT NORTHSIDE BAPTIST CHURCH ON 2·6·2005

I would like to first of all explain that to remember what to say I have to use notes. In preparing to speak about Stewardship I asked God to lead me and give me the words to say in order to speak to those of you who are not tithing, for whatever reason you might have, let me start with a brief history of who I am and where I came from, I was born in a small town in Illinois, I was one of 8 children, my mother was married 3 times, as we were growing up our family was very poor. My grandfather on my mother's side was killed in a car/train accident before I was born, and my grandfather on my father's side was killed in a refinery accident when I was 2 years old, I. Mentioned earlier that my mother had been married 3 times, her second husband was my father, my parents were divorced when I was 3 years old, my father had a serious drinking problem, after my parents divorced even though my father lived within 10 miles from me, I have only seen him 7 or 8 times my entire life, most of my memories of my family were after my mother married her third husband who was 20 years older then her (he died of cancer when I was 18 years old) I have 2 older sisters who both dropped out of school and were married after becoming pregnant. My 2 older brothers were both always in trouble, in and out of jail from the time they were 16 years old. I realize now that God had to be looking out for me or I would of never had a chance in life. Our family never discussed God and went to Church only 2 or 3 times my entire childhood. I still remember a couple of times my stepfather slammed the door on visiting Preachers!! well I made it through those years and thru Walmart I was able to do ok in life, but I still did not know God, after Ramona and I were married we went to Church occasionally and I began to learn a little about religion and Church life, over the years as we moved with Walmart we would go to Church occasionally, only for Worship service, I have to tell you that I was listening but all I heard was words, then one fall day in 1995 our family was out for a ride in the country when we passed by a Church that stood on a hill, then the event that would change my family's life forever happened my youngest son looked up at the Church and said Daddy what does that T stand for? God spoke to me that very minute and told me that I needed to get and keep my family in Church, so we went to the Church that my son had pointed to and started going every week, I had a new commitment to learn for myself what that T stood for, we had a very good Preacher who told it like it is, each week I felt the Lord telling me to accept him as my Savior, but I was stubborn and resisted, then in December of 1996 one of my department managers at Walmart gave me this poem (Read it now) I was immediately convicted and made the decision to accept the Lord, that Sunday 12-15-1996 I walked down the aisle and accepted Jesus as my Savior, the Bible says that Jesus will save whosoever asks him to, if you do not know Jesus as your Savior, time is running out, accept him now before it is everlasting too late.

TWAS THE NIGHT BEFORE
JESUS CAME

Twas the night before Jesus came and all through the house,
Not a creature was praying, not one in the house.
Their Bibles were lain on the shelf without care,
In hopes that Jesus would not come there.

The children were dressing to crawl into bed,
Not once ever kneeling or bowing a head.
And Mom in the rocker with Baby on her lap,
Was watching the Late Show while I took a nap.

When out of the East there arose such a clatter,
I sprang to my feet to see what was the matter.
Away to the window I flew like a flash!
Tore open the shutters and threw up the sash!

When what to my wondering eyes should appear,
But angels proclaiming that Jesus was here!
With a light like the sun sending forth a bright ray,
I knew in a moment this must be the day.

The light of his face made me cover my heard,
It was Jesus returning just like he said.
And though I possessed worldly wisdom and wealth,
I cried when I saw him in spite of myself.

In The Book of Life which he held in his hand,
Was written the name of every saved man.
He spoke not a word as he searched for my name,
When he said "It's not here." My head hung in shame.

The people whose names had been written with love,
He gathered to take to his Father above.
With those who were ready he arose without a sound,
While all the rest were left standing around.

I fell to my knees, but it was too late,
I had waited too long and thus sealed my fate.
I stood and I cried as they arose out of sight,
Oh, if only I had been ready tonight!

In the words of this poem the meaning is clear,
The coming of Jesus is drawing near.
There's only one life and when comes the last call,
We'll find that the Bible was true after all!

The Sunday after I was saved our Pastor preached from Malachi 3 verses 7-11 (read now) I wanted to be obedient to God's command so I started to tithe 10% of my pay, the next Sunday our Pastor said he needed to clarify that the 10 % needed to come off the top he said that the taxes, social security etc was between us and the Government, God wants us to give him the first 10 % and do it cheerfully.

I thought to myself what is he going to ask for next Sunday? But I wanted to do what God commanded so I started tithing 10 % off the top, I continued to tithe and to go to Church and learned more about God's word including his promises such as Luke 6 verse 38 (read now) the Pastor said we could never out give God.

After we started tithing things changed for my family, things we had wanted to do (but always had stumbling blocks in our way) finally started happening I'll give you a few examples.

1. we were in Virginia and wanted to move back closer to home Ramona Kentucky and Richard Illinois but after trying several times to transfer with Walmart we basically gave up on moving back home.

2. So we decided we would stay in Virginia, we loved our Church and our Pastor, we had decided to buy a house the following year in 1999 when all of a sudden, in March of 1998 our landlord decided to move back to our house, we had 60 days to move out. (if you are ever in that position you do not feel like you are about to be blessed) so we figured we would just go ahead and buy a house a little earlier then we had planned on. It sounded like a good plan except nothing worked out, there was not very much housing available in the first place and our son Samuel had school and neighbor friends and wanted to go to the same school they did which limited our area to find a house in.

Time was moving on and we were faced with a date to move out so we did what we should have done first, we prayed and asked God to lead us and we agreed together to follow God's will.

I don't remember exactly why I did it but I looked at the stores that Walmart had available and Columbia Tennessee was available so I applied for that store, it was such a long shot I didn't even tell Ramona I had applied for it at the time.

A couple of weeks went by, 37 store managers had applied for the Columbia store. They told me that I was in the top 5, then I told Ramona that I had applied, obviously I did get the Columbia store.

Then we faced a new challenge we had to move to Columbia in a couple weeks, we had only a short time left to be in the Virginia house and I had to begin working at the Columbia Walmart very soon, so we made a trip down to Columbia 2 weeks before we were going to move there, to find a house to rent. We looked all weekend (no luck) everything was to small or rented out, Ramona called the last person on our list about a four bedroom house, the lady didn't answer, we were very discouraged, we hadn't found a place to live and we would be moving to Columbia in 2 weeks. We were out of options so we headed out of town and back towards home, then Ramona's purse started talking. Hello Hello, without the phone ringing, the last person Ramona had called was on the phone, she had a house in the country to rent and wanted us to come over and see it, we rented the house and moved to Columbia. When I agreed to take the Columbia store, I took a pay cut of 15 % because we had been living in a town close to Washington DC and Walmart pays a premium if you live close to a city. It was worth the pay cut to get closer to home my wife's parents were not in great shape and we wanted to be closer to them. When we finished 1998 and the store's profits were figured out (I receive a small percentage as a bonus) the Columbia store had created a Bonus for me of exactly the same amount above the old store as I had lost by going to Columbia, in other words I had came out even in pay, even though I had planned on a 15 % pay cut.

I am 100 % convinced that God blessed our family for being faithful and tithing like he commanded us to do.

I would like to leave you with just a thought, as parents God trusts us to raise our Children to fear him and to serve in his Kingdom, I think that this is the most important thing any of us will ever do, our job is getting tougher every day the devil is on the throne in this world and it becomes more evil every day, Paul warned us of this in Second Timothy Chapter 3 verses 1-4 Read now.

Paul also wrote the answer for us, what we need to do as parents to train our Children, in Second Timothy Chapter 3 verses 14-17.

What Paul is saying is to teach our Children God's word, as a person who grew up without God I can tell you that I missed out on a lot I would encourage every parent here to bring your Children to Church every time the doors are open, Sunday School, Worship Service, Discipleship training and Wednesday night RA and GA, let's give our Children these 5 hours a week in God's house.

In closing I would like to urge anyone who is here today that if you are not tithing, take God at his word start tithing and just see how your life will change and what blessings God will shower you with.

Thank you and may God bless you.

MY TESTIMONY GIVEN AT NORTHSIDE BAPTIST CHURCH ON 2-19-2006

Good morning

Today I will be talking about stewardship which is not just about money it is more about God's will for our lives.

Last Sunday our pastor gave his testimony about his life and growing up in a Christian home, unfortunately my childhood was much different.

My mother was married 3 times, her second husband was my father, they were divorced when I was 3. I have 2 older brothers both were in and out of jail my entire childhood, I have 2 older sisters both become pregnant and left home at young ages. Growing up my family didn't talk about God and we went to Church only a handful of times, even though I did not know God, he was still looking out for me and putting things in front of me that would lead me to his son Jesus.

First of all he lead me to Kentucky where I would meet and marry Ramona, who came from a Christian family. After we were married we started to go to Church on an irregular basis, Sunday worship service only. The second part of God's plan for my Salvation came in late 1995, we had lived In Manassas Virginia for a little more than 4 years, as we headed west of town on a road trip to see the mountains that we could only barely see from our home, it was a beautiful fall day the leaves were beginning to turn colors and the scenery was amazing as we past a Church that stood on a hill, my Son Samuel who was 8 years old pointed to that Church and asked Daddy what does that T stand for?

Ramona explained to Samuel that the T stood for the cross that Jesus had died on, I cannot explain the horrible feeling that both me and Ramona felt at that very moment, I thought how can my 8 year old son not know about Jesus, then I realized that I really didn't know either, well I knew that something was missing in my life and that little question that Samuel raised shook my world.

Ramona and I decided to go and visit that Church where Samuel had asked that important question (Daddy what does that T stand for?)

so we started going to Battlefield Baptist Church, we both liked the Church something was different about it to me it seemed more serious, more real and of course there was Preacher Karl Skinner, how do I describe this man, he was a man about 50 years old rather short nearly bald and kind of chunky I never ever heard someone preach like he did, he said the words like he actually meant and believed them he was animated, he jumped up and down he was positive and enthusiastic Whow!

We went to this Church every Sunday for worship service the entire family went sometimes willingly sometimes not so willingly but we all went and soon we started talking about God and Samuel and the rest of us learned about Jesus and what that T stands for, it became normal to go to Church.

Every week I understood more about the Church and what it is all about, every week during the invitation our Pastor Karl Skinner pleaded with those of us who didn't know Jesus to accept his free gift of Salvation, at first I thought it was a waste of time how could just going up to the front of the Church talking to the preacher do anything?

Well as the weeks went by I began to understand because as the preacher was talking, I began to feel something inside of me telling me that I was lost and needed the Lord, each Sunday the tug on my heart become stronger and stronger, I realized that it was just a matter of time before I would have to make a decision but every Sunday I would resist and come up with reasons in my head why it shouldn't be this week.

That was when God sealed the deal and sent a message that I would finally get.

While I was doing my job working at Walmart in the middle of the Christmas season, It happened, one of my department managers said Richard read this poem it is really good, this is the poem I read that day (read poem now)

TWAS THE NIGHT BEFORE
JESUS CAME

Twas the night before Jesus came and all through the house,
Not a creature was praying, not one in the house.
Their Bibles were lain on the shelf without care,
In hopes that Jesus would not come there.

The children were dressing to crawl into bed,
Not once ever kneeling or bowing a head.
And Mom in the rocker with Baby on her lap,
Was watching the Late Show while I took a nap.

When out of the East there arose such a clatter,
I sprang to my feet to see what was the matter.
Away to the window I flew like a flash!
Tore open the shutters and threw up the sash!

When what to my wondering eyes should appear,
But angels proclaiming that Jesus was here!
With a light like the sun sending forth a bright ray,
I knew in a moment this must be the day.

The light of his face made me cover my heard,
It was Jesus returning just like he said.
And though I possessed worldly wisdom and wealth,
I cried when I saw him in spite of myself.

In The Book of Life which he held in his hand,
Was written the name of every saved man.
He spoke not a word as he searched for my name,
When he said "It's not here." My head hung in shame.

The people whose names had been written with love,
He gathered to take to his Father above.
With those who were ready he arose without a sound,
While all the rest were left standing around.

I fell to my knees, but it was too late,
I had waited too long and thus sealed my fate.
I stood and I cried as they arose out of sight,
Oh, if only I had been ready tonight!

In the words of this poem the meaning is clear,
The coming of Jesus is drawing near.
There's only one life and when comes the last call,
We'll find that the Bible was true after all!

I read this poem and I was immediately overpowered with the Holy Spirit telling me to quit stalling and to accept the offer of Salvation, I had no choice, I made the decision to be Saved that coming Sunday. Sunday 12-15-1996 came and I announced to my family that morning before Church that I had made the decision and would go down the aisle, I did this in advance to set an example for my Children.

When we got to Church, I could not tell you what the pastor Skinner's message was, I could only think about getting down the aisle and getting Saved.

When the invitation came I went down the aisle and accepted the Lord Jesus Christ as my personal Savior. The same day 12-15-1996 I was Baptized, I then had the inner peace that I had been searching for all of my life.

I would like to take a minute and talk to anyone who is here today and is not Saved. Like I have told you I was not raised in a Christian home and was not Saved until I was 35. I was very stubborn and was hard to convince that I needed Jesus, God gave me chance after chance and put things in my path to lead me to Jesus, thankfully I finally got smart and accepted the free gift of Salvation.

Today I would ask you a couple of questions

#1 why are you here today? Is it an accident, a co-incidence or is it God that put you here today?

#2 think back and see if God has put you in contact with Christians who told you about Jesus, Was it an accident or co-incidence or is it God put you in the right place at the right time?

#3 once I awakened and knew that I was headed for hell all I could think of was that I was going to send my Children to hell because I would not accept Jesus as my Savior, because I knew that I have influence on my family and what I do, they are likely to do, so I ask you? Where are you leading your Children Grandchildren and family?

If nothing else gets you to accept the Lord, do it because what you do makes a difference in your family.

Brother John Buchanan gave us all a great example, it does not matter your age or position in life if you are not Saved make the decision today, answer that tug on your heart and accept the Lord to I would like to site some scripture references to speak to this fact.

Luke 19 verses 1-10 read now
Acts 11 verse 14 read now
Acts 16 verses 26-33 read now
Acts 18 verse 8 read now

Just like the scriptures show can happen, after I was Saved every one of my Children accepted the Lord and were Saved Praise God!!

This is Stewardship month so I want to talk about what God expects from us once we are Saved, again I will use my own experiences to explain how God honors his words.

The Sunday after I was saved our Pastor preached from Malachi 3 verses 7-11 (read now) I wanted to be obedient to God's command so I started to tithe 10% of my pay, the next Sunday our Pastor said he needed to clarify that the 10 % needed to come off the top he said that the taxes, social security etc was between us and the Government, God wants us to give him the first 10 % and do it cheerfully.

I thought to myself what is he going to ask for next Sunday? But I wanted to do what God commanded so I started tithing 10 % off the top, I continued to tithe and to go to Church and learned more about God's word including his promises such as Luke 6 verse 38 (read now) the Pastor said we could never out give God.

After we started tithing things changed for my family, things we had wanted to do (but always had stumbling blocks in our way) finally started happening I'll give you a few examples.

1. we were in Virginia and wanted to move back closer to home Ramona Kentucky and Richard Illinois but after trying several times to transfer with Walmart we basically gave up on moving back home.
2. So we decided we would stay in Virginia, we loved our Church and our Pastor, we had decided to buy a house the following year in 1999 when all of a sudden, in March of 1998 our landlord decided to move back to our house, we had 60 days to move out. (if you are ever in that position you do not feel like you are

about to be blessed) so we figured we would just go ahead and buy a house a little earlier then we had planned on. It sounded like a good plan except nothing worked out, there was not very much housing available in the first place and our son Samuel had school and neighbor friends and wanted to go to the same school they did which limited our area to find a house in.

Time was moving on and we were faced with a date to move out so we did what we should have done first, we prayed and asked God to lead us and we agreed together to follow God's will.

I don't remember exactly why I did it but I looked at the stores that Walmart had available and Columbia Tennessee was available so I applied for that store, it was such a long shot I didn't even tell Ramona I had applied for it at the time.

A couple of weeks went by, 37 store managers had applied for the Columbia store. They told me that I was in the top 5, then I told Ramona that I had applied, obviously I did get the Columbia store.

Then we faced a new challenge we had to move to Columbia in a couple weeks, we had only a short time left to be in the Virginia house and I had to begin working at the Columbia Walmart very soon, so we made a trip down to Columbia 2 weeks before we were going to move there, to find a house to rent. We looked all weekend (no luck) everything was to small or rented out, Ramona called the last person on our list about a four bedroom house, the lady didn't answer, we were very discouraged, we hadn't found a place to live and we would be moving to Columbia in 2 weeks. We were out of options so we headed out of town and back towards home, then Ramona's purse started talking. Hello Hello, without the phone ringing, the last person Ramona had called was on the phone, she had a house in the country to rent and wanted us to come over and see it, we rented the house and moved to Columbia. When I agreed to take the Columbia store, I took a pay cut of 15 % because we had been living in a town close to Washington DC and Walmart pays a premium if you live close to a city. It was worth the pay cut to get closer to home my wife's parents were not in great shape and we wanted to be closer to them. When we finished 1998 and the store's profits were figured out (I receive a small percentage as a bonus) the Columbia store had created a Bonus for me of exactly the same amount above the old store as I had lost by going to Columbia, in other words I had came out even in pay, even though I had planned on a 15% pay cut.

I am 100% convinced that God blessed our family for being faithful and tithing like he commanded us to do.

I would like to leave you with just a thought, as parents God trusts us to raise our Children to fear him and to serve in his Kingdom, I think that this is the most important thing any of us will ever do, our job is getting tougher every day the devil is on the throne in this world and it becomes more evil every day Paul warned us of this in Second Timothy Chapter 3 verses 1-4 Read now

Paul also wrote the answer for us, what we need to do as parents to train our Children, in Second Timothy Chapter 3 verses 14-17.

What Paul is saying is to teach our Children God's word, as a person who grew up without God I can tell you that I missed out on a lot I would encourage every parent here to bring your Children to Church every time the doors are open, Sunday School, Worship Service, Discipleship training and Wednesday night RA and GA, let's give our Children these 5 hours a week in God's house.

I will leave you with a couple of thoughts

First
Listen for God, he will nudge you into following his will for your life if you let him, I have already give you some examples of how he has lead me.

1. marrying Ramona
2. the day Samuel asked about the cross
3. the day my associate gave me the poem
4. our lease being canceled and not able to find a house
5. Columbia Tennessee Walmart coming available at the correct time

Two other things I will tell you about I hadn't mentioned earlier

#1 after I started tithing we were to get a tax refund and I did not know weather to tithe on it or not, after talking it over with Ramona and praying about it I decided to err on the side of giving more to God since I was not sure if I should tithe on it or not.

Within three weeks of tithing on that tax refund I received in the mail a check from the IRS of exactly the amount I had tithed on the earlier tax refund, along with a note saying I had made an error on the taxes and the note said that the IRS would send a letter explaining what mistake I had made.

To this date I have not received an explanation from the IRS but I know in my heart that it was God blessing me for tithing on that tax refund.

#2 the second thing I haven't spoke about is my family coming to this Church.

When we first came to Columbia we went to every Baptist Church in Columbia some twice, I can tell you that this Church is special, the first time we came here you could feel the Holy Spirit moving and the Congregation made us feel welcome the very first day, but we were not convinced until the second time we came here, the Preacher said one sentence that we had heard our last Preacher say every week. Pastor

Rushing said we must keep the main thing the main thing, at that moment me and Ramona knew that God had lead us to this Church.

Within a few months the Sunday school Director and his family moved out of town, and the Pastor asked me if I would be Sunday School Director, remember I had been Saved less then 2 years and I had no clue of even what a Sunday School Director even does.

But I prayed about it and the Lord told me to do it, so I accepted the position.

I can tell you that our Pastor is a man of God and if he asks you to do something you can count on it being something that God wants you to do.

Someone recently asked me if I would ever go to another Church and I explained to them that God brought me and my family to this Church and only God will send me anywhere else.

The last thing that I will say is be bold for God, listen to what he is saying and just do it, I will use my Daughter Katie as an example to follow.

On Katie's first week of high school, her freshman year, she was in science class and got into a discussion about God and how to be Saved and Katie lead a fellow student to the Lord in the middle of science class.

Then in the last Revival Katie was troubled about a little girl that she had befriended several years ago when the girl was 5 or 6, the Preacher was Preaching about hell and not letting your family or friends go there, Katie had told the little girl about hell and how to be Saved years ago, but after that their parents stopped letting her play with Katie and she lost track of her.

In that Revival meeting Katie told me and Ramona that she had to go and talk to that girl now!!, of course we first thought of how late it was and how it might appear, knocking on someone's door at 9 pm on a Wednesday night, but Katie would have none of it, she was determined to go and talk to her little friend and save her from hell, so after Revival I took Katie to the house the girl had lived in, we expected to see the girl and her parents come to the door instead this 50 plus year old man with a New Jersey accent came to the door.

Katie asked the man where the little girl was and the man said that the family had moved 6 months ago and that he now lived there, I thought well that is it let's go home but Katie had no intention of giving up she told the man about Revival and that she had been told to go to this house tonight because someone there needed the Lord and she didn't want anyone to go to hell.

He along with me were both amazed, he said young lady you have got the wrong house and she said if you die today will you go to Heaven or hell?

Are you Saved?

He said I am probably not Saved like you think Saved means but I have been to a Church before. Katie continued and thru her own tears told him that Jesus loved him and didn't want him to go to hell, she told him the plan of Salvation.

He stood there and listened with great interest in what she said, he then turned Katie away.

She invited him to Revival and told him that she would Pray for him

I do not know if that man has been Saved but I do know that Katie did her part in sharing Jesus and God's word will eventually bear fruit.

I am 44 years old and that was the bravest thing I have ever seen, I am very proud of Katie she gives us big brave adults an example of being bold for God.

Thank you and may God bless you!

MY TESTIMONY AT
NORTHSIDE BAPTIST CHURCH
GIVEN ON 3-22-2009

I want to talk to you today about Stewardship, in the times we find ourselves in.

The Bible tells us how we are to react to what is going on in the world, I would ask you to turn in your Bible to 1st Peter Chapter 4 verses 4-10 I will read it now. Our Pastor tells us that no one can take away your personal Testimony and what God has done for you, so I will share with you how God helped me through a trying situation, maybe this will help someone here who may go through a trial in life.

Some of you may remember in the fall of 2006, it was all over the news about how Walmart who I worked for, was supporting the homosexual lifestyle, as many of my fellow Christians this deeply concerned me to the point that I considered leaving the company, I thought that if I worked for a company that supported this type of behavior I would be a part of it, and reflect poorly on my Savior. The news came out right before our fall Walmart store managers meeting, I had prayed about the situation and asked God to guide me, before the meeting I had prepared a couple of letters to Walmart Executives.

1. Lee Scott CEO
2. Rob Walton Majority owner of Walmart

I felt lead to take a stand at our Walmart meeting against our company supporting this type of behavior and I really thought that I would of good conscience have to leave Walmart.

The following is my account of what happened at that meeting.

On the morning of 9-10-2006, I went to Walmart's Chapel service. During this service I talked to God and asked him to lead me and if it was his will for me to take a stand for him at Walmart, I asked him to put the CEO of Walmart Lee Scott in my path so that I could speak to him. I really wanted not to see Lee Scott, it would have been easier for me just to mail the

letter I had prepared for him and the Chairman of the Board of Walmart Rob Walton, after I had returned home.

On Sunday 9-10-2006 at 2pm I nearly walked into the CEO of Walmart Lee Scott, I took one look at him and thought to myself oh no!! That instant I knew that God had put Lee Scott in my path so I said to myself hello Richard this is it, you either stand up for what you believe or chicken out and regret it the rest of your life. As I approached Lee, the 4 or 5 people that were around him left and it was just him and me so I took a deep breath and went up to Lee, I handed him the envelope that contained the letter that I had earlier prepared for him. He took the envelope and looked at me, I said Lee this is a letter that I wrote you, please read it when you can, then I got braver and I said, what this is about is Walmart supporting the National gay and lesbian group, Lee said Walmart is not supporting that group, I said there has been a press release from the group saying that Walmart is a member and there has been newspaper articles saying the same thing. Lee said what happened is that a low level home office associate who is gay joined the national gay and lesbian group by himself, not on behalf of Walmart. Then the national gay and lesbian group immediately sent out a press release stating that Walmart is a member of and supports their group, he said this is not true he also said we will not pay for same sex partner health insurance benefits.

I then said that if that is the case then Walmart needs to correct the record and let the public know that we do not support that group Lee said that Walmart had decided not to say anything, they preferred just to let the issue die. I told Lee that I didn't want to tell him how to do his job but this is a big deal, that it had upset Christians that Walmart would support such a group and that local preachers were passing out copies of the national gay and lesbian group's press release and were preaching against shopping at Walmart. In addition to that, I have had lots of people calling me and telling me in person that they were concerned about Walmart supporting this group and that they would stop shopping at Walmart. Lee said that Walmart was in the middle of a lot of issues like plan b abortion

pill and immigration and that Walmart could not win either way, he said that the whole Walmart supporting the gay and lesbian group issue would blow over in a couple of weeks. I told Lee that I personally was concerned about this and that I would suggest that he set the record straight. Lee said that he didn't want to appear that we were anti gay or against any group, I told Lee that Jesus said that we should love everyone. I added that even though we should love everyone, we should not support something that God is against, Lee said I guess God will sort it out after we die. Lee left and went his way.

After my discussion with the CEO of Walmart, God gave me an amazing peace about the situation.

I know that as Christians in this world we will be faced with bad situations and will have to make choices, I hope this example will provide some hope for someone going through a challenging situation Thank you and may God bless you

This is a picture that I sent (along with my letter) to Lee Scott and Rob Walton, the picture is of me and Sam Walton that was taken in 1981 when Sam Walton visited the Walmart store in Taylorville Illinois.

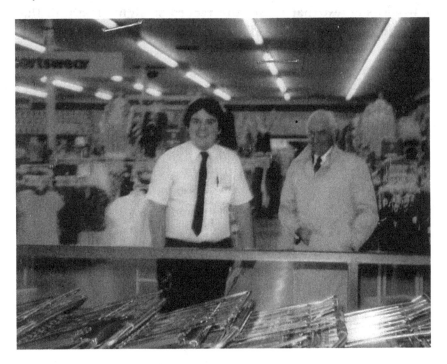

Dear Mr. Rob Walton and Mr. Lee Scott,

My name is Richard Baud and I am currently the Store Manager of Columbia Tennessee Wal-Mart.

I am writing to you because of the announcement by Wal-Mart that our company has recently made a $25,000 contribution to the NGLCC (National Gay & Lesbian Chamber of Commerce) and Wal-Mart has now developed a partnership with this group.

The reason that I chose to write to both of you is simply that you have the power to either make or seriously influence decisions that affect every associate and every member of management that works for our company.

I started my career with Wal-Mart at age 19 on 12-30-80 and I have been a loyal Wal-Mart employee over these many years working hard along with my co-workers to help build our company. Shortly after I began with Wal-Mart I was assigned to the Taylorville, IL store as Assistant Manager. There in early 1982 had my first in person meeting with our founder Sam Walton. As Sam Walton normally did he met with our management team after he toured our store. It was at that meeting in our snack bar that Sam asked me which company I had worked for prior to Wal-Mart and why I had left them. During our discussion I told him that my previous company treated people badly and their executives took kickbacks from vendors and at corporate functions hard liquor was served. Then Sam Walton told me that I had made a good choice at coming to Wal-Mart. Sam said that he and his family believed in the golden rule – Do unto others as you would have them do unto you. Sam said that Wal-Mart would always use the Good Book – The Bible, as its guide in its dealings.

I have always been proud of our company taking a stand, for example when Wal-Mart edited music and took out materials that were unfit to be sold in a Wal-Mart store.

I am not sure how Wal-Mart made the decision to publicly and proudly proclaim its partnership with this organization, but I do know that this puts Wal-Mart on the wrong side of the Bible and what God finds acceptable.

You two gentlemen have a huge responsibility in leading a giant like Wal-Mart; millions of people, Wal-Mart associates, vendors, and customers depend on Wal-Mart and Wal-Mart due to its size and success is a leader. Many companies will follow Wal-Mart's lead and go down the same path.

I respectfully am asking for you two leaders to stand up for what is morally right and reverse this decision and return Wal-Mart back to where our founder Sam Walton left it A moral leader in our nation where our associates can be proud to work and our customers can be proud to shop.

I realize that I am only one person and that my voice is weak but I pray that you both will take my request into consideration. I believe that Wal-Mart has been richly blessed by God over the years and by turning away from God Wal-Mart will no longer enjoy these blessings.

Thank you for reading and considering my request,

May God Bless You,

Richard Baud
9-8-06

MY TESTIMONY GIVEN AT NORTHSIDE BAPTIST CHURCH ON 9-4-2011

Good morning, please excuse me for reading this but if I don't write it down I cannot remember details very well.

The reason I am up here this morning is to give credit where credit is due.

On 7-24-2011 my mom died after a 6 year battle with cancer, over these last 6 years our Church has had my mom on our Prayer list and many kind words have been expressed and get well cards sent.

A special thank you for Lois Lindsey, she sent my mom tons of cards and letters and they meant so much to my mom, on behalf of my family thank you.

Pastor John Rushing always said that people can debate lots of things but they cannot take away your personal testimony, so I will make this as quick as I can but you need to know how God has answered prayers and worked miracles.

I know that most of you grew up in Church and have lived the Christian life all of your lives, this was not the case with my family, my mother was a good woman she worked hard and did whatever she had to, to raise me and my 7 brothers and sisters, but she made lots of mistakes and bad decisions in her life, my mother was pregnant at 17 years old and married the father, she divorced twice and married 3 times, my father was her second husband.

We grew up not going to Church with no talk about God.

Through a series of God working in my life I was saved on 12-15-1996, since that day my biggest priority has been to see my family saved, God has worked in my immediate family and all of my Children have accepted the Lord, since I was saved I have reached out to my extended family including my mother and brothers and sisters witnessing to them and praying every day for their Salvation.

This is a tough crowd and all of my attempts have failed, most of my siblings ignored me and their was some comments about me being one of those religious fanatics, then my mother got sick and our Church started praying for her.

Very gradually she began to listen to what I had to say about the Lord, and I know that she was touched by the kind words from Lois Lindsey.

I once thought it was sad that my mother had to get sick to warm up to the Gospel but now I know it took that to wake her up, as my mother got sicker she realized her death was coming and she finally realized she needed Jesus, I had several discussions with my mother about her Salvation and I thought she had been Saved but I was not sure.

So I prayed to God that he would give me one more chance to be sure she was Saved, I asked God to allow me some time alone with her and that she would be alert and receptive to the plan of Salvation.

I went to see my mom in the hospital on Friday night 7-15-2011, when I got there my mom was alone and alert, we had a nice talk and she brought up the fact that she was probably not going to get better and did not think she would live much longer, she said she was ready to be with God, I asked her if she was sure about her Salvation she was not sure so I asked her if I could share God's plan of Salvation with her, she asked me to, I used the Roman Road and shared God's plan of Salvation with her.

I read Romans 3 verse 23
I read Romans 5 verse 8
I read Romans 6 verse 23
I read Romans 10 verses 9 and 10
I read Romans 10 verse 13

THE ROMAN ROAD

Jesus prepared for us a simple plan of salvation. Presented in the Book of Romans of the Holy Bible, this outline will show you step by step how to be saved.

ROMANS 3:23
"For all have sinned, and come short of the glory of God." —— ALL have sinned ——

ROMANS 5:8
"But God commendeth his love toward us, in that, while we were yet sinners, Christ died for us" —— ALL are loved ——

ROMANS 6:23
"For the wages of sin is death, but the gift of God is eternal life through Jesus Christ our Lord." —— The PAYMENT for sin is death, separation from God forever But salvation is a GIFT from God, not earned by going to church, baptism, good works, etc. ——

ROMANS 10:9, 10
"That if thou shalt confess with thy mouth the Lord Jesus, and shalt believe in thine heart that God hath raised him from the dead, THOU SHALT BE SAVED." "For with the heart man believeth unto righteousness; and with the mouth confession is made unto salvation." —— Just BELIEVE and RECEIVE ——

ROMANS 10:13
*For WHOSOEVER shall can upon the name of the Lord SHALL BE SAVED."

AFTER FOLLOWING THE PLAN OF
SALVATION LEAD THEM IN THIS PRAYER

Dear Lord Jesus, I'm a Sinner —— I'm Lost. I Need to be Saved. I Want to be Saved. If You Will Save Me, I'll Give You My Life. Thank You Jesus for Saving Me.

**—— After praying this prayer, go over the scriptures
on the other side of this card ——**

My mom accepted the Lord as her Savior at 1030 pm that night Praise the Lord!

After my mother passed away on Sunday 7-24-2011, I asked God to give me peace about my mother, on the way home from Illinois I turned the radio on to a Gospel station, the very first words I heard from that song was (she is in a better place)

God is good!

My mother is in Heaven and I am not worried about her any more, but I am concerned about my brothers and sisters who are not Saved.

I spoke to Pastor Ron and let him know my extended family members were not Saved and I asked him to pray for their Salvation I know that you all have been praying for them.

I spoke to the Pastor that did my mother's funeral, the day before her funeral, he had worked with her for 10 years (before she retired) at the local Hershey's candy factory, I asked him if he had ever asked my mother about her Salvation (he had not) I told him about her Salvation experience and I asked him to use the funeral to witness to my family members who might be more receptive to the message if they knew my mom had accepted the Lord, he was a little hesitant but said he would.

God heard your prayers, at my moms Funeral that Preacher preached a Sermon, he said during his Sermon that he had been up since 3 am wrestling with what he would say, he could not rest.

During his Sermon he was very direct

First he said that my mother had gambled with her eternal life to the last minute.

Second he said that if they ever wanted to see my mom again they would need to follow her example and accept the Lord as their personal Savior, he shared the plan of Salvation.

Third he spoke of Jesus and how God sent him to die for our sins.

I could see people around the room listening carefully I believe that, that Sermon will lead to great things for my family over the years.

Again thank you, please keep my family in your prayers.

I want to encourage everyone who has a family member not saved, don't give up it took 15 and a half years from the day I was saved for my mother to be saved.

Also if you are here today and you are not saved, I want you to listen carefully to me, I was 35 before I accepted the Lord as my personal Savior, I was in Church for years before then sitting week after week listening to the Preacher, I understood about Jesus and about the Bible but I knew I was not saved, if that is you this morning make today the day you make the decision to step out on faith and accept Jesus as your Savior.

We are not promised tomorrow don't gamble with your eternal life.

As I close I would like to share something else with you, my mother did not have it easy in life and made some difficult decisions.

When she was 17 she was pregnant and chose to keep the baby and get married, when I was 2 years old my mother divorced my father who was a drunk, at that time she had 6 children then she found out she was pregnant with # 7, she gave that child up for adoption providing a family that could not have a child an awesome blessing, she could have made another bad choice and aborted her baby.

Many women today are finding themselves in simulator situations you can help.

The Pregnancy Center of Columbia is conducting a drive to get 1000 people to sign up for a monthly auto draft of $10, this is a small enough amount to enable most people to afford it and if 1000 people sign up for it, it would pay most of the Center's expenses that will enable the Center to help people like my mother in their time of need make a good choice.

So I am asking you to take one of the forms that will be available after Church this morning and fill it out and be a Partner with our Pregnancy Center.

Thank you and may God bless you.

Our Pastor has asked me to lead our prayer, if you feel lead to to come to the Alter please do.

My prayer, thank you for allowing us in your house today, forgive us for our sins, be with our prayers this morning, heal the sick, comfort the grieving.

Father I ask that you would touch the hearts of anyone here today and is not saved, I pray that they would not leave this place today until they have accepted the free gift of Salvation, be with our Pastor and give him words to say, Lord we ask that as we begin our new Church year that you will lead guide and direct each activity of our Church, in Jesus name I pray

Amen.

After this Testimony Betty Smith, who was a Sunday School Teacher for 4-5 year olds (while I was Sunday School Director) came to me and told me that on that night 7-15-2011 she woke up from a dream where she was told to pray for my mother, so she prayed for my mom and her Salvation at the very time mom accepted the Lord.

Praise God

Chapter / Northside Baptist Church

I thank God for Northside Baptist Church and the awesome people who have attended and served at this Church over the years.

CHAPTER 8

MY PHILOSOPHY

I n this chapter I will layout my core beliefs, these beliefs have been learned from 60 years of life starting with my Childhood growing up poor and continuing with my career in retail and with my religious journey leading to my Salvation thru Jesus Christ and what I have learned from being a Father and Grandfather.

I will start with I believe about the Country that I have been blessed to have been born in and lived all my life.

Godly people came to America wanting to be free to Worship God.

Our founders were wise enough to set up our Country with With God's word as the guiding principles, if God does not make the rules who does?

How do we decide what is right or wrong?

Our system of Government only works when our Citizens follow Godly Principles, our Country will only succeed with Citizens who are Moral and Decent.

Our founders set up our Government with checks and balances and the ability of our people to correct mistakes in the form of Amending the Constitution, the basic goodness of God fearing people, has been able to correct many mistakes over the years using these Amendments.

Our freedom would not be possible without our people stepping up to serve and protect our Country, without these brave men and women fighting and dying for our Country we would not still be free.

I believe that America's prosperity comes from God and the strong work ethic that his people have. What allows America to work is that we allow normal people (regardless of their background) to benefit from their labors ideas and imagination.

Without taxing it all away from them, there are lots of examples around the world where common people cannot benefit from their dreams.

The belief that the Government owns you and all that you do, dooms those Countries to mediocrity. These Countries are where the dreamers come from that want to migrate to America, our immigration policy should be able to encourage these folks to come to America to live out their Dreams.

On politics I consider myself a Christian Conservative who leans towards the Libertarian point of view letting the individual make decisions that are best for them and their families. I believe that our political leaders should help guide their people to do what is just and right. But today a significant portion of our political leaders simply follow the path of least resistance making decisions based on how to get reelected with no concern of how their decisions will effect their voters long term interests including spending money we do not have on programs that will not help them, help themselves but get them more dependent on Government and run up debt that our Grandkids will be cursed with.

On Community, I believe that a significant portion of our Community Leaders are leading their Communities to ruin by rabble rousing and spreading division based on race, economic status and Religion. Focusing on trying to get easy money for their people from Government instead of helping their folks become self-reliant and raise their Children to become self-reliant, some of our Community leaders choose to tear down those in their Community that are self-reliant instead of using them as positive examples for their folks to emulate.

I believe that the way to solve local problems like

1. homelessness
2. poverty
3. drug and alcohol addiction
4. children that grow up without the support of a good family

Are best resolved by local folks coming together to fix those problems thru Churches, Charitable organizations, and local Governments.

If all of these resources (both human and financial) will come together these problems can be improved upon.

With my background of having managed Walmart stores I can clearly say that a good family behind you will help you succeed, for the most part those who succeed at a job have a support system such as Family, Friends, Church. I have seen this truth in every Walmart that I have managed, I have seen many hard working people fail because they lack a good support system, if your car breaks down if you have a support system, someone will drive you to work or help get your car fixed.

Many times folks that do not have this support will end up losing their job due to lack of good transportation to and from work, there are many other situations that people find themselves in that requires assistance at times for an example your babysitter doesn't make it and you are unable to get to work, if you have a family member or a friend that can watch your children then you can make it to work if you don't have that support, this can lead to you losing your job.

I also believe that Christians need to vote every single time, in the primaries and general elections for local State and National Elections, and be an educated voter voting for leaders that will lead our Country back to God.

In closing this Chapter I have attached copies of the following founding documents, The Declaration of Independence, The Constitution including The Bill of rights and the Amendments to the Constitution and The Federalist Papers (due to the size of these papers I have only added the topics not the entire articles), please take the time to read them, many politicians refer to a small part of one of these documents that fit into their own political view, but they sometimes will take it out of context, now you can read the entire document and hold your leaders accountable to vote to uphold our values.

"PREAMBLE" OF THE
DECLARATION OF INDEPENDENCE

We hold these truths to be self-evident, that all men are created equal, that they are endowed by their Creator with certain unalienable Rights, that among these are Life, Liberty and the pursuit of Happiness. That to secure these rights, Governments are instituted among Men, deriving their just powers from the consent of the governed. That whenever any Form of Government becomes destructive of these ends, it is the Right of the People to alter or to abolish it, and to institute new Government, laying its foundation on such principles and organizing its powers in such form, as to them shall seem most likely to effect their Safety and Happiness. Prudence, indeed, will dictate that Governments long established should not be changed for light and transient causes; and accordingly all experience hath shown that mankind are more disposed to suffer, while evils are sufferable, than to right themselves by abolishing the forms to which they are accustomed. But when a long train of abuses and usurpations, pursuing invariably the same Object evinces a design to reduce them under absolute Despotism, it is their right, it is their duty, to throw off such Government, and to provide new Guards for their future security.

DECLARATION OF INDEPENDENCE: A TRANSCRIPTION

Note: The following text is o transcription of the Stone Engraving of the parchment Declaration of Independence (the document on display in the Rotunda at the National Archives Museum.) The spelling and punctuation reflects the original.

In Congress, July 4, 1776

The unanimous Declaration of the thirteen united States of America, When in the Course of human events, it becomes necessary for one people to dissolve the political bands which have connected them with another, and to assume among the powers of the earth, the separate and equal station to which the Laws of Nature and of Nature's God entitle them, a decent respect to the opinions of mankind requires that they should declare the causes which impel them to the separation.

We hold these truths to be self-evident, that all men are created equal, that they are endowed by their Creator with certain unalienable Rights, that among these are Life, Liberty and the pursuit of Happiness.--That to secure these rights, Governments are instituted among Men, deriving their just powers from the consent of the governed, --That whenever any Form of Government becomes destructive of these ends, it is the Right of the People to alter orto abolish it, and to institute new Government, laying its foundation on such principles and organizing its powers in such form, as to them shall seem most likely to effect their Safety and Happiness. Prudence, indeed, will dictate that Governments long established should not be changed for light and transient causes; and accordingly all experience hath shewn, that mankind are more disposed to suffer, while evils are sufferable, than to right themselves by abolishing the forms to which they are accustomed. But when a long train of abuses and usurpations, pursuing invariably the same Object evinces a design to reduce them under absolute Despotism, it is their right, it is their duty, to throw off such Government, and to provide new Guards for their future security.--Such has been the patient sufferance of these Colonies; and such is now the necessity which constrains them to alter their former Systems of Government. The history of the present King of Great Britain is a history of repeated injuries and usurpations, all having in direct object the establishment of an absolute Tyranny over these States. To prove this, let Facts be submitted to a candid world.

He has refused his Assent to Laws, the most wholesome and necessary for the public good.

He has forbidden his Governors to pass Laws of immediate and pressing importance, unless suspended in their operation till his Assent should be obtained; and when so suspended, he has utterly neglected to attend to them.

He has refused to pass other Laws for the accommodation of large districts of people, unless those people would relinquish the right of Representation in the Legislature, a right inestimable to them and formidable to tyrants only.

He has called together legislative bodies at places unusual, uncomfortable, and distant from the depository of their public Records, for the sole purpose of fatiguing them into compliance with his measures.

He has dissolved Representative Houses repeatedly, for opposing with manly firmness his invasions on the rights of the people.

He has refused for a long time, after such dissolutions, to cause others to be elected; whereby the Legislative powers, incapable of Annihilation, have returned to the People at large for their exercise; the State remaining in the mean time exposed to all the dangers of invasion from without, and convulsions within.

He has endeavoured to prevent the population of these States; for that purpose obstructing the Laws for Naturalization of Foreigners; refusing to pass others to encourage their migrations hither, and raising the conditions of new Appropriations of Lands.

He has obstructed the Administration of Justice, by refusing his Assent to Laws for establishing Judiciary powers.

He has made Judges dependent on his Will alone, for the tenure of their offices, and the amount and payment of their salaries.

He has erected a multitude of New Offices, and sent hither swarms of Officers to harrass our people, and eat out their substance.

He has kept among us, in times of peace, Standing Armies without the Consent of our legislatures.

He has affected to render the Military independent of and superior to the Civil power.

He has combined with others to subject us to a jurisdiction foreign to our constitution, and unacknowledged by our laws; giving his Assent to their Acts of pretended Legislation:

For Quartering large bodies of armed troops among us:

For protecting them, by a mock Trial, from punishment for any Murders which they should commit on the Inhabitants of these States:

For cutting off our Trade with all parts of the world:

For imposing Taxes on us without our Consent:

For depriving us in many cases, of the benefits of Trial by Jury:

For transporting us beyond Seas to be tried for pretended offences

For abolishing the free System of English Laws in a neighbouring Province, establishing therein an Arbitrary government, and enlarging its Boundaries so as to render it at once an example and fit instrument for introducing the same absolute rule into these Colonies:

For taking away our Charters, abolishing our most valuable Laws, and altering fundamentally the Forms of our Governments:

For suspending our own Legislatures, and declaring themselves invested with power to legislate for us in all cases whatsoever.

He has abdicated Government here, by declaring us out of his Protection and waging War against us.

He has plundered our seas, ravaged our Coasts, burnt our towns, and destroyed the lives of our people.

He is at this time transporting large Armies of foreign Mercenaries to compleat the works of death, desolation and tyranny, already begun with circumstances of Cruelty & perfidy scarcely paralleled in the most barbarous ages, and totally unworthy the Head of a civilized nation.

He has constrained our fellow Citizens taken Captive on the high Seas to bear Arms against their Country, to become the executioners of their friends and Brethren, or to fall themselves by their Hands.

He has excited domestic insurrections amongst us, and has endeavoured to bring on the inhabitants of our frontiers, the merciless Indian Savages, whose known rule of warfare, is an undistinguished destruction of all ages, sexes and conditions.

In every stage of these Oppressions We have Petitioned for Redress in the most humble terms: Our repeated Petitions have been answered only by repeated injury. A Prince whose character is thus marked by every act which may define a Tyrant, is unfit to be the ruler of a free people.

Nor have We been wanting in attentions to our British brethren. We have warned them from time to time of attempts by their legislature to extend an unwarrantable jurisdiction over us. We have reminded them of the circumstances of our emigration and settlement here. We have appealed to their native justice and magnanimity, and we have conjured them by the ties of our common kindred to disavow these usurpations, which, would inevitably interrupt our connections and correspondence. They too have been deaf to the voice of justice and of consanguinity. We must, therefore, acquiesce in the necessity, which denounces our Separation, and hold them, as we hold the rest of mankind, Enemies in War, in Peace Friends.

We, therefore, the Representatives of the united States of America, in General Congress, Assembled, appealing to the Supreme Judge of the world for the rectitude of our intentions, do, in the Name, and by Authority of the good People of these Colonies, solemnly publish and declare, That these United Colonies are, and of Right ought to be Free and Independent States; that they are Absolved from all Allegiance to the British Crown, and that all political connection between them and the State of Great Britain, is and ought to be totally dissolved; and that as Free and Independent States, they have full Power to levy War, conclude Peace, contract Alliances, establish Commerce, and to do all other Acts and Things which Independent States may of right do. And for the support of this Declaration, with a firm reliance on the protection of divine Providence, we mutually pledge to each other our Lives, our Fortunes and our sacred Honor.

Georgia
Button Gwinnett
Lyman Hall
George Walton

North Carolina
William Hooper
Joseph Hewes
John Pennsylvania

South Carolina
Edward Rutledge
Thomas Heyward, Jr.
Thomas Lynch, Jr.
Arthur Middleton

Massachusetts
John Hancock

Maryland
Samuel Chase
William Paca
Thomas Stone
Charles Carroll of Carrollton

Virginia
George Wythe
Richard Henry Lee
Thomas Jefferson
Benjamin Harrison
Thomas Nelson, Jr.
Francis Lightfoot Lee
Carter Braxton

Pennsylvania
Robert Morris
Benjamin Rush
Benjamin Franklin
John Morton
George Clymer
James Smith
George Taylor
James Wilson
George Ross

Delaware
Caesar Rodney
George Read
Thomas McKean

New York
William Floyd
Philip Livingston

Francis Lewis
Lewis Morris

New Jersey
Richard Stockton
John Witherspoon
Francis Hopkinson
John Hart
Abraham Clark

New Hampshire
Josiah Bartlett
William Whipple

Massachusetts
Samuel Adams
John Adams
Robert Treat Paine
Elbridge Gerry

Rhode Island
Stephen Hopkins
William Ellery

Connecticut
Roger Sherman
Samuel Huntington
William Williams
Oliver Wolcott

New Hampshire
Matthew Thornton

THE CONSTITUTION OF THE UNITED STATES: A TRANSCRIPTION

Note: The following text is a transcription of the Constitution as it was inscribed by Jacob Shallus on parchment (the document on display in the Rotunda at the National Archives Museum.) *The spelling and punctuation reflect the original.*

We the People of the United States, in Order to form a more perfect Union, establish Justice, insure domestic Tranquility, provide for the common defence, promote the general Welfare, and secure the Blessings of Liberty to ourselves and our Posterity, do ordain and establish this Constitution for the United States of America.

Article. I.

Section, 1.

All legislative Powers herein granted shall be vested in a Congress of the United States, which shall consist of a Senate and House of Representatives.

Section. 2.

The House of Representatives shall be composed of Members chosen every second Year by the People of the several States, and the Electors in each State shall have the Qualifications requisite for Electors of the most numerous Branch of the State Legislature.

No Person shall be a Representative who shall not have attained to the Age of twenty five Years, and been seven Years a Citizen of the United States, and who shall not, when elected, be an Inhabitant of that State in which he shall be chosen.

Representatives and direct Taxes shall be apportioned among the several States which may be included within this Union, according to their respective Numbers, which shall be determined by adding to the whole Number of free Persons, including those bound to Service for a Term of Years, and excluding Indians not taxed, three fifths of all other Persons. The actual Enumeration shall be made within three Years after the first Meeting of the Congress of the United States, and within every subsequent Term often Years, in such Manner as they shall by Law direct. The Number of Representatives shall not exceed one for every thirty Thousand, but each State shall have at Least one Representative; and until such enumeration shall be made, the State of New Hampshire shall be entitled to chuse three, Massachusetts eight, Rhode-Island and Providence Plantations one, Connecticut five, New-York six, New Jersey four, Pennsylvania eight, Delaware one, Maryland six, Virginia ten, North Carolina five, South Carolina five, and Georgia three.

When vacancies happen in the Representation from any State, the Executive Authority thereof shall issue Writs of Election to fill such Vacancies.

The House of Representatives shall chuse their Speaker and other Officers; and shall have the sole Power of Impeachment.

Section. 3.

The Senate of the United States shall be composed of two Senators from each State, chosen by the Legislature thereof, for six Years; and each Senator shall have one Vote.

Immediately after they shall be assembled in Consequence of the first Election, they shall be divided as equally as may be into three Classes. The Seats of the Senators of the first Class shall be vacated at the Expiration of the second Year, of the second Class at the Expiration of the fourth Year, and of the third Class at the Expiration of the sixth Year, so that one third may be chosen every second Year; and if Vacancies happen by Resignation, or otherwise, during the Recess of the Legislature of any State, the Executive thereof may make temporary

Appointments until the next Meeting of the Legislature, which shall then fill such Vacancies.

No Person shall be a Senator who shall not have attained to the Age of thirty Years, and been nine Years a Citizen of the United States, and who shall not, when elected, be an Inhabitant of that State for which he shall be chosen.

The Vice President of the United States shall be President of the Senate, but shall have noVote, unless they be equally divided.

The Senate shall chuse their other Officers, and also a President pro tempore, in the Absence of the Vice President, or when he shall exercise the Office of President of the United States.

The Senate shall have the sole Power to try all Impeachments. When sitting for that Purpose, they shall be on Oath or Affirmation. When the President of the United States is tried, the Chief Justice shall preside: And no Person shall be convicted without the Concurrence of two thirds of the Members present.

Judgment in Cases of Impeachment shall not extend further than to removal from Office, and disqualification to hold and enjoy any Office of honor, Trust or Profit under the United States: but the Party convicted shall nevertheless be liable and subject to Indictment, Trial, Judgment and Punishment, according to Law.

Section. 4.

The Times, Places and Manner of holding Elections for Senators and Representatives, shall be prescribed in each State by the Legislature thereof; but the Congress may at any time by Law make or alter such Regulations, except as to the Places of chusing Senators.

The Congress shall assemble at least once in every Year, and such Meeting shall be on the first Monday in December, unless they shall by Law appoint a different Day.

Section. 5.

Each House shall be the Judge of the Elections, Returns and Qualifications of its own Members, and a Majority of each shall constitute a Quorum to do Business; but a smaller Number may adjourn from day to day, and may be authorized to compel the Attendance of absent Members, in such Manner, and under such Penalties as each House may provide.

Each House may determine the Rules of its Proceedings, punish its Members for disorderly Behaviour, and, with the Concurrence of two thirds, expel a Member.

Each House shall keep a Journal of its Proceedings, and from time to time publish the same, excepting such Parts as may in their Judgment require Secrecy; and the Yeas and Nays of the Members of either House on any question shall, at the Desire of one fifth of those Present, be entered on the Journal.

Neither House, during the Session of Congress, shall, without the Consent of the other, adjourn for more than three days, nor to any other Place than that in which the two Houses shall be sitting.

Section. 6.

The Senators and Representatives shall receive a Compensation for their Services, to be ascertained by Law, and paid out of the Treasury of the United States. They shall in all Cases, except Treason, Felony and Breach of the Peace, be privileged from Arrest during their Attendance at the Session of their respective Houses, and in going to and returning from the same; and for any Speech or Debate in either House, they shall not be questioned in any other Place.

No Senator or Representative shall, during the Time for which he was elected, be appointed to any civil Office under the Authority of the United States, which shall have been created, or the Emoluments whereof shall have been encreased during such time; and no Person holding any Office under the United States, shall be a Member of either House during his Continuance in Office.

Section. 7.

All Bills for raising Revenue shall originate in the House of Representatives; but the Senate may propose or concur with Amendments as on other Bills.

Every Bill which shall have passed the House of Representatives and the Senate, shall, before it become a Law, be presented to the President of the United States; If he approve he shall sign it, but if not he shall return it, with his Objections to that House in which it shall have originated, who shall enter the Objections at large on their Journal, and proceed to reconsider it. If after such Reconsideration two thirds of that House shall agree to pass the Bill, it shall be sent, together with the Objections, to the other House, by which it shall likewise be reconsidered, and if approved by two thirds of that House, it shall become a Law. But in all such Cases the Votes of both Houses shall be determined by yeas and Nays, and the Names of the Persons voting for and against the Bill shall be entered on the Journal of each House respectively. If any Bill shall not be returned by the President within ten Days (Sundays excepted) after it shall have been presented to him, the Same shall be a Law, in like Manner as if he had signed it, unless the Congress by their Adjournment prevent its Return, in which Case it shall not be a Law.

Every Order, Resolution, or Vote to which the Concurrence of the Senate and House of Representatives may be necessary (except on a question of Adjournment) shall be presented to the President of the United States; and before the Same shall take Effect, shall be approved by him, or being disapproved by him, shall be repassed by two thirds of the Senate and House of Representatives, according to the Rules and Limitations prescribed in the Case of a Bill.

Section. 8.

The Congress shall have Power To lay and collect Taxes, Duties, Imposts and Excises, to pay the Debts and provide for the common Defence and general Welfare of the United States; but all Duties, Imposts and Excises shall be uniform throughout the United States;

To borrow Money on the credit of the United States;

To regulate Commerce with foreign Nations, and among the several States, and with the Indian Tribes;

To establish an uniform Rule of Naturalization, and uniform Laws on the subject of Bankruptcies throughout the United States;

To coin Money, regulate the Value thereof, and of foreign Coin, and fix the Standard of Weights and Measures;

To provide for the Punishment of counterfeiting the Securities and current Coin of the United States;

To establish Post Offices and post Roads;

To promote the Progress of Science and useful Arts, by securing for limited Times to Authors and Inventors the exclusive Right to their respective Writings and Discoveries;

To constitute Tribunals inferior to the supreme Court;

To define and punish Piracies and Felonies committed on the high Seas, and Offences against the Law of Nations;

To declare War, grant Letters of Marque and Reprisal, and make Rules concerning Captures on Land and Water;

To raise and support Armies, but no Appropriation of Money to that Use shall be for a longer Term than two Years;

To provide and maintain a Navy;

To make Rules for the Government and Regulation of the land and naval Forces;

To provide for calling forth the Militia to execute the Laws of the Union, suppress Insurrections and repel Invasions;

To provide for organizing, arming, and disciplining, the Militia, and for governing such Part of them as may be employed in the Service of the United States, reserving to the States respectively, the Appointment of the Officers, and the Authority of training the Militia according to the discipline prescribed by Congress;

To exercise exclusive Legislation in all Cases whatsoever, over such District (not exceeding ten Miles square) as may, by Cession of particular States, and the Acceptance of Congress, become the Seat of the Government of the United States, and to exercise like Authority overall Places purchased by the Consent of the Legislature of the State in which the Same shall be, for the Erection of Forts, Magazines, Arsenals, dock-Yards, and other needful Buildings;——And

To make all Laws which shall be necessary and proper for carrying into Execution the foregoing Powers, and all other Powers vested by this Constitution in the Government of the United States, or in any Department or Officer thereof.

Section. 9.

The Migration or Importation of such Persons as any of the States now existing shall think proper to admit, shall not be prohibited by the Congress prior to the Year one thousand eight hundred and eight, but a Tax or duty may be imposed on such Importation, not exceeding ten dollars for each Person.

The Privilege of the Writ of Habeas Corpus shall not be suspended, unless when in Cases of Rebellion or Invasion the public Safety may require it.

No Bill of Attainder or ex post facto Law shall be passed.

No Capitation, or other direct, Tax shall be laid, unless in Proportion to the Census or enumeration herein before directed to be taken.

No Tax or Duty shall be laid on Articles exported from any State.

No Preference shall be given by any Regulation of Commerce or Revenue to the Ports of one State over those of another: nor shall Vessels bound to, or from, one State, be obliged to enter, clear, or pay Duties in another.

No Money shall be drawn from the Treasury, but in Consequence of Appropriations made by Law; and a regular Statement and Account of the Receipts and Expenditures of all public Money shall be published from time to time.

No Title of Nobility shall be granted by the United States: And no Person holding any Office of Profit or Trust under them, shall, without the Consent of the Congress, accept of any present, Emolument, Office, or Title, of any kind whatever, from any King, Prince, or foreign State.

Section. 10.

No State shall enter into any Treaty, Alliance, or Confederation; grant Letters of Marque and Reprisal; coin Money; emit Bills of Credit; make any Thing but gold and silver Coin a Tender in Payment of Debts; pass any Bill of Attainder, ex post facto Law, or Law impairing the Obligation of Contracts, or grant any Title of Nobility.

No State shall, without the Consent of the Congress, lay any Imposts or Duties on Imports or Exports, except what may be absolutely necessary for executing it's inspection Laws: and the net Produce of all Duties and Imposts, laid by any State on Imports or Exports, shall be for the Use of the Treasury of the United States; and all such Laws shall be subject to the Revision and Controul of the Congress.

No State shall, without the Consent of Congress, lay any Duty of Tonnage, keep Troops, or Ships of War in time of Peace, enter into any Agreement or Compact with another State, or with a foreign Power, or engage in War, unless actually invaded, or in such imminent Danger as will not admit of delay.

Article. II.

Section, 1.

The executive Power shall be vested in a President of the United States of America. He shall hold his Office during the Term of four Years, and, together with the Vice President, chosen for the same Term, be elected, as follows

Each State shall appoint, in such Manner as the Legislature thereof may direct, a Number of Electors, equal to the whole Number of Senators and Representatives to which the State may be entitled in the Congress: but no Senator or Representative, or Person holding an Office of Trust or Profit under the United States, shall be appointed an Elector.

The Electors shall meet in their respective States, and vote by Ballot for two Persons, of whom one at least shall not be an Inhabitant of the same State with themselves. And they shall make a List of all the Persons voted for, and of the Number of Votes for each; which List they shall sign and certify, and transmit sealed to the Seat of the Government of the United States, directed to the President of the Senate. The President of the Senate shall, in the Presence of the Senate and House of Representatives, open all the Certificates, and the Votes shall then be counted. The Person having the greatest Number of Votes shall be the President, if such Number be a Majority of the whole Number of Electors appointed; and if there be more than one who have such Majority, and have an equal Number of Votes, then the House of Representatives shall immediately chuse by Ballot one of them for President; and if no Person have a Majority, then from the five highest on the List the said House shall in like Manner chuse the President. But in chusing the President, the Votes shall be taken by States, the Representation from each State having one Vote; A quorum for this Purpose shall consist of a Member or Members from two thirds of the States, and a Majority of all the States shall be necessary to a Choice. In every Case, after the Choice of the President, the Person having the greatest Number of Votes of the Electors shall be the Vice President. But if there should remain two or more who have equal Votes, the Senate shall chuse from them by Ballot the Vice President.

The Congress may determine the Time of chusing the Electors, and the Day on which they shall give their Votes; which Day shall be the same throughout the United States.

No Person except a natural born Citizen, or a Citizen of the United States, at the time of the Adoption of this Constitution, shall be eligible to the Office of President; neither shall any Person be eligible to that Office who shall not have attained to the Age of thirty five Years, and been fourteen Years a Resident within the United States.

In Case of the Removal of the President from Office, or of his Death, Resignation, or Inability to discharge the Powers and Duties of the said Office, the Same shall devolve on the Vice President, and the Congress may by Law provide for the Case of Removal, Death, Resignation or Inability, both of the President and Vice President, declaring what Officer shall then act as President, and such Officer shall act accordingly, until the Disability be removed, or a President shall be elected.

The President shall, at stated Times, receive for his Services, a Compensation, which shall neither be encreased nor diminished during the Period for which he shall have been elected, and he shall not receive within that Period any other Emolument from the United States, or any of them.

Before he enter on the Execution of his Office, he shall take the following Oath or Affirmation:——"I do solemnly swear (or affirm) that I will faithfully execute the Office of President of the United States, and will to the best of my Ability, preserve, protect and defend the Constitution of the United States."

Section. 2.

The President shall be Commander in Chief of the Army and Navy of the United States, and of the Militia of the several States, when called into the actual Service of the United States; he may require the Opinion, in writing, of the principal Officer in each of the executive Departments, upon any Subject relating to the Duties of their respective Offices, and he shall have Power to grant Reprieves and Pardons for Offences against the United States, except in Cases of Impeachment.

He shall have Power, by and with the Advice and Consent of the Senate, to make Treaties, provided two thirds of the Senators present concur; and he shall nominate, and by and with the Advice and Consent of the Senate, shall appoint Ambassadors, other public Ministers and Consuls, Judges of the supreme Court, and all other Officers of the United States, whose Appointments are not herein otherwise provided for, and which shall be established by Law: but the Congress may by Law vest the Appointment of such inferior Officers, as they think proper, in the President alone, in the Courts of Law, or in the Heads of Departments.

The President shall have Power to fill up all Vacancies that may happen during the Recess of the Senate, by granting Commissions which shall expire at the End of their next Session.

Section. 3.

He shall from time to time give to the Congress Information of the State of the Union, and recommend to their Consideration such Measures as he shall judge necessary and expedient; he may, on extraordinary Occasions, convene both Houses, or either of them, and in Case of Disagreement between them, with Respect to the Time of Adjournment, he may adjourn them to such Time as he shall think proper; he shall receive Ambassadors and other public Ministers; he shall take Care that the Laws be faithfully executed, and shall Commission all the Officers of the United States.

Section. 4.

The President, Vice President and all civil Officers of the United States, shall be removed from Office on Impeachment for, and Conviction of, Treason, Bribery, or other high Crimes and Misdemeanors.

Article III.

Section. 1.

The judicial Power of the United States, shall be vested in one supreme Court, and in such inferior Courts as the Congress may from time to time ordain and establish. The Judges, both of the supreme and inferior Courts, shall hold their Offices during good Behaviour, and shall, at stated Times, receive for their Services, a Compensation, which shall not be diminished during their Continuance in Office.

Section. 2.

The judicial Power shall extend to all Cases, in Law and Equity, arising under this Constitution, the Laws of the United States, and Treaties made, or which shall be made, under their Authority; —to all Cases affecting Ambassadors, other public Ministers and Consuls;—to all Cases of admiralty and maritime Jurisdiction;—to Controversies to which the United States shall be a Party;—to Controversies between two or more States;— between a State and Citizens of another State,—between Citizens of different States,—between Citizens of the same State claiming Lands under Grants of different States, and between a State, or the Citizens thereof, and foreign States, Citizens or Subjects.

In all Cases affecting Ambassadors, other public Ministers and Consuls, and those in which a State shall be Party, the supreme Court shall have original Jurisdiction. In all the other Cases before mentioned, the supreme Court shall have appellate Jurisdiction, both as to Law and Fact, with such Exceptions, and under such Regulations as the Congress shall make.

The Trial of all Crimes, except in Cases of Impeachment, shall be by Jury; and such Trial shall be held in the State where the said Crimes shall have been committed; but when not committed within any State, the Trial shall be at such Place or Places as the Congress may by Law have directed.

Section. 3.

Treason against the United States, shall consist only in levying War against them, or in adhering to their Enemies, giving them Aid and Comfort. No Person shall be convicted of Treason unless on the Testimony of two Witnesses to the same overt Act, or on Confession in open Court.

The Congress shall have Power to declare the Punishment of Treason, but no Attainder of Treason shall work Corruption of Blood, or Forfeiture except during the Life of the Person attainted.

Article. IV.

Section, 1.

Full Faith and Credit shall be given in each State to the public Acts, Records, and judicial Proceedings of every other State. And the Congress may by general Laws prescribe the Manner in which such Acts, Records and Proceedings shall be proved, and the Effect thereof.

Section. 2.

The Citizens of each State shall be entitled to all Privileges and Immunities of Citizens in the several States.

A Person charged in any State with Treason, Felony, or other Crime, who shall flee from Justice, and be found in another State, shall on Demand of the executive Authority of the State from which he fled, be delivered up, to be removed to the State having Jurisdiction of the Crime.

No Person held to Service or Labour in one State, under the Laws thereof, escaping into another, shall, in Consequence of any Law or Regulation therein, be discharged from such Service or Labour, but shall be delivered up on Claim of the Party to whom such Service or Labour may be due.

Section. 3.

New States may be admitted by the Congress into this Union; but no new State shall be formed or erected within the Jurisdiction of any other State; nor any State be formed by the Junction of two or more States, or Parts of States, without the Consent of the Legislatures of the States concerned as well as of the Congress.

The Congress shall have Power to dispose of and make all needful Rules and Regulations respecting the Territory or other Property belonging to the United States; and nothing in this Constitution shall be so construed as to Prejudice any Claims of the United States, or of any particular State.

Section. 4.

The United States shall guarantee to every State in this Union a Republican Form of Government, and shall protect each of them against Invasion; and on Application of the Legislature, or of the Executive (when the Legislature cannot be convened) against domestic Violence.

Article. V.

The Congress, whenever two thirds of both Houses shall deem it necessary, shall propose Amendments to this Constitution, or, on the Application of the Legislatures of two thirds of the several States, shall call a Convention for proposing Amendments, which, in either Case, shall be valid to all Intents and Purposes, as Part of this Constitution, when ratified by the Legislatures of three fourths of the several States, or by Conventions in three fourths thereof, as the one or the other Mode of Ratification may be proposed by the Congress; Provided that no Amendment which may be made prior to the Year One thousand eight hundred and eight shall in any Manner affect the first and fourth Clauses in the Ninth Section of the first Article; and that no State, without its Consent, shall be deprived of its equal Suffrage in the Senate.

Article. VI.

All Debts contracted and Engagements entered into, before the Adoption of this Constitution, shall be as valid against the United States under this Constitution's under the Confederation.

This Constitution, and the Laws of the United States which shall be made in Pursuance thereof; and all Treaties made, or which shall be made, under the Authority of the United States, shall be the supreme Law of the Land; and the Judges in every State shall be bound thereby, any Thing in the Constitution or Laws of any State to the Contrary notwithstanding.

The Senators and Representatives before mentioned, and the Members of the several State Legislatures, and all executive and judicial Officers, both of the United States and of the several States, shall be bound by Oath or Affirmation, to support this Constitution; but no religious Test shall ever be required as a Qualification to any Office or public Trust under the United States.

Article. VII.

The Ratification of the Conventions of nine States, shall be sufficient for the Establishment of this Constitution between the States so ratifying the Same.

The Word, "the," being interlined between the seventh and eighth Lines of the first Page, The Word "Thirty" being partly written on an Erazure in the fifteenth Line of the first Page, The Words "is tried" being interlined between the thirty second and thirty third Lines of the first Page and the Word "the" being interlined between the forty third and forty fourth Lines of the second Page.

Attest William Jackson Secretary

done in Convention by the Unanimous Consent of the States present
the Seventeenth Day of September in the Year of our Lord one thousand
seven hundred and Eighty seven and of the Independance of the United
States of America the Twelfth In witness whereof We have hereunto
subscribed our Names,

G°. Washington
Presidt and deputy from Virginia

Delaware

Geo: Read
Gunning Bedford
jun
John Dickinson
Richard Bassett
Jaco: Broom

Maryland

James McHenry
Dan of St Thos.
Jenifer
Danl. Carroll

Virginia

John Blair
James Madison Jr.

North Carolina

Wm. Blount
Richd. Dobbs
Spaight
Hu Williamson

South Carolina

J. Rutledge
Charles Cotesworth
Pinckney
Charles Pinckney
Pierce Butler

Georgia

William Few
Abr Baldwin

New Hampshire

John Langdon
Nicholas Gilman

Massachusetts

Nathaniel Gorham
Rufus King

Connecticut

Wm. Saml.
Johnson
Roger Sherman

New York

Alexander
Hamilton

New Jersey

Wil: Livingston
David Brearley
Wm. Paterson
Jona: Dayton

Pennsylvania

B Franklin
Thomas Mifflin
Robt. Morris
Geo. Clymer
Thos. FitzSimons
Jared Ingersoll
James Wilson
Gouv Morris

For biographies of the non-signing delegates to the Constitutional Convention, see the Founding Fathers page.

he Bill of Rights: A Transcription

Note: The following text is a transcription of the enrolled original of the Joint Resolution of Congress proposing the Bill of Rights, which is on permanent display in the Rotunda at the National Archives Museum. The spelling and punctuation reflects the original.

On September 25, 1789, the First Congress of the United States proposed 12 amendments to the Constitution. The 1789 Joint Resolution of Congress proposing the amendments is on display in the Rotunda in the National Archives Museum. Ten of the proposed 12 amendments were ratified by three-fourths of the state legislatures on December 15, 1791. The ratified Articles (Articles 3-12) constitute the first 10 amendments of the Constitution, or the U.S. Bill of Rights. In 1992, 203 years after it was proposed, Article 2 was ratified as the 27th Amendment to the Constitution. Article 1 was never ratified.

Transcription of the 1789 Joint Resolution of Congress Proposing 12 Amendments to the U.S. Constitution

Congress of the United States begun and held at the City of New-York, on Wednesday the fourth of March, one thousand seven hundred and eighty nine.

THE Conventions of a number of the States, having at the time of their adopting the Constitution, expressed a desire, in order to prevent misconstruction or abuse of its powers, that further declaratory and restrictive clauses should be added: And as extending the ground of public confidence in the Government, will best ensure the beneficent ends of its institution.

RESOLVED by the Senate and House of Representatives of the United States of America, in Congress assembled, two thirds of both Houses concurring, that the following Articles be proposed to the Legislatures of the several States, as amendments to the Constitution of the United States, all, or any of which Articles, when ratified by three fourths of the said Legislatures, to be valid to all intents and purposes, as part of the said Constitution; viz.

ARTICLES in addition to, and Amendment of the Constitution of the United States of America, proposed by Congress, and ratified by the Legislatures of the several States, pursuant to the fifth Article of the original Constitution.

Article the first... After the first enumeration required by the first article of the Constitution, there shall be one Representative for every thirty thousand, until the number shall amount to one hundred, after which the proportion shall be so regulated by Congress, that there shall be not less than one hundred Representatives, nor less than one Representative for every forty thousand persons, until the number of Representatives shall amount to two hundred; after which the proportion shall be so regulated by Congress, that there shall not be less than two hundred Representatives, nor more than one Representative for every fifty thousand persons.

Article the second... No law, varying the compensation for the services of the Senators and Representatives, shall take effect, until an election of Representatives shall have intervened.

Article the third... Congress shall make no law respecting an establishment of religion, or prohibiting the free exercise thereof; or abridging the freedom of speech, or of the press; or the right of the people peaceably to assemble, and to petition the Government for a redress of grievances.

Article the fourth... A well regulated Militia, being necessary to the security of a free State, the right of the people to keep and bear Arms, shall not be infringed.

Article the fifth... No Soldier shall, in time of peace be quartered in any house, without the consent of the Owner, nor in time of war, but in a manner to be prescribed by law.

Article the sixth... The right of the people to be secure in their persons, houses, papers, and effects, against unreasonable searches and seizures, shall not be violated, and no Warrants shall issue, but upon probable cause, supported by Oath or affirmation, and particularly describing the place to be searched, and the persons or things to be seized.

Article the seventh... No person shall be held to answer for a capital, or otherwise infamous crime, unless on a presentment or indictment of a Grand Jury, except in cases arising in the land or naval forces, or in the Militia, when in actual service in time of War or public danger; nor shall any person be subject for the same offence to be twice put in jeopardy of life or limb; nor shall be compelled in any criminal case to be a witness against himself, nor be deprived of life, liberty, or property, without due process of law; nor shall private property be taken for public use, without just compensation.

Article the eighth... In all criminal prosecutions, the accused shall enjoy the right to a speedy and public trial, by an impartial jury of the State and district wherein the crime shall have been committed, which district shall have been previously ascertained by law, and to be informed of the nature and cause of the accusation; to be confronted with the witnesses against him; to have compulsory process for obtaining witnesses in his favor, and to have the Assistance of Counsel for his defence.

Article the ninth... In suits at common law, where the value in controversy shall exceed twenty dollars, the right of trial by jury shall be preserved, and no fact tried by a jury, shall be otherwise re-examined in any Court of the United States, than according to the rules of the common law.

Article the tenth... Excessive bail shall not be required, nor excessive fines imposed, nor cruel and unusual punishments inflicted.

Article the eleventh... The enumeration in the Constitution, of certain rights, shall not be construed to deny or disparage others retained by the people.

Article the twelfth... The powers not delegated to the United States by the Constitution, nor prohibited by it to the States, are reserved to the States respectively, or to the people.

ATTEST,

Frederick Augustus Muhlenberg, Speaker of the House of Representatives
John Adams, Vice-President of the United States, and President of the Senate
John Beckley, Clerk of the House of Representatives.
Sam. A Otis Secretary of the Senate

The U.S. Bill of Rights

Note: The following text is a transcription of the first ten amendments to the Constitution in their original form. These amendments were ratified December 15, 1791, and form what is known as the "Bill of Rights."

Amendment I

Congress shall make no law respecting an establishment of religion, or prohibiting the free exercise thereof; or abridging the freedom of speech, or of the press; or the right of the people peaceably to assemble, and to petition the Government for a redress of grievances.

Amendment II

A well regulated Militia, being necessary to the security of a free State, the right of the people to keep and bear Arms, shall not be infringed.

Amendment III

No Soldier shall, in time of peace be quartered in any house, without the consent of the Owner, nor in time of war, but in a manner to be prescribed by law.

Amendment IV

The right of the people to be secure in their persons, houses, papers, and effects, against unreasonable searches and seizures, shall not be violated, and no Warrants shall issue, but upon probable cause, supported by Oath or affirmation, and particularly describing the place to be searched, and the persons or things to be seized.

Amendment V

No person shall be held to answer for a capital, or otherwise infamous crime, unless on a presentment or indictment of a Grand Jury, except in cases arising in the land or naval forces, or in the Militia, when in actual service in time of War or public danger; nor shall any person be subject for the same offence to be twice put in jeopardy of life or limb; nor shall be compelled in any criminal case to be a witness against himself, nor be deprived of life, liberty, or property, without due process of law; nor shall private property be taken for public use, without just compensation.

Amendment VI

In all criminal prosecutions, the accused shall enjoy the right to a speedy and public trial, by an impartial jury of the State and district wherein the crime shall have been committed, which district shall have been previously ascertained by law, and to be informed of the nature and cause of the accusation; to be confronted with the witnesses against him; to have compulsory process for obtaining witnesses in his favor, and to have the Assistance of Counsel for his defence.

Amendment VII

In Suits at common law, where the value in controversy shall exceed twenty dollars, the right of trial by jury shall be preserved, and no fact tried by a jury, shall be otherwise re-examined in any Court of the United States, than according to the rules of the common law.

Amendment VIII

Excessive bail shall not be required, nor excessive fines imposed, nor cruel and unusual punishments inflicted.

Amendment IX

The enumeration in the Constitution, of certain rights, shall not be construed to deny or disparage others retained by the people.

Amendment X

The powers not delegated to the United States by the Constitution, nor prohibited by it to the States, are reserved to the States respectively, or to the people.

Note: The capitalization and punctuation in this version is from the enrolled original of the Joint Resolution of Congress proposing the Bill of Rights, which is on permanent display in the Rotunda of the National Archives Building, Washington, D.C.

The Constitution: Amendments 11-27

Constitutional Amendments 1-10 make up what is known as The Bill of Rights. Amendments 11-27 are listed below.

AMENDMENT XI

Passed by Congress March 4, 1794. Ratified February 7, 1795.

Note: Article III, section 2, of the Constitution was modified by amendment 11. The Judicial power of the United States shall not be construed to extend to any suit in law or equity, commenced or prosecuted against one of the United States by Citizens of another State, or by Citizens or Subjects of any Foreign State.

AMENDMENT XII

Passed by Congress December 9, 1803. Ratified June 15, 1804.

Note: A portion of Article II, section 1 of the Constitution was superseded by the 12th amendment. The Electors shall meet in their respective states and vote by ballot for President and Vice-President, one of whom, at least, shall not be an inhabitant of the same state with themselves; they shall name in their ballots the person voted for as President, and in distinct ballots the person voted for as Vice-President, and they shall make distinct lists of all persons voted for as President, and of all persons voted for as Vice-President, and of the number of votes for each, which lists they shall sign and certify, and transmit sealed to the seat of the government of the United States, directed to the President of the Senate; -- the President of the Senate shall, in the presence of the Senate and House of Representatives, open all the certificates and the votes shall then be counted; -- The person having the greatest number of votes for President, shall be the President, if such number be a majority of the whole number of Electors appointed; and if no person have such majority, then from the persons having the highest numbers not exceeding three on the list of those voted for as President, the House of Representatives shall choose immediately, by ballot, the President. But in choosing the President, the votes shall be taken by states, the representation from each state having one vote; a quorum for this purpose shall consist of a member or members from two-thirds of the states, and a majority of all the states shall be necessary to a choice. [And if the House of Representatives shall not choose a President whenever the right of choice shall devolve upon them, before the fourth day of March next following, then the Vice-President shall act as President, as in case of the death or other constitutional disability of the President. --]* The person having the greatest number of votes as Vice-President, shall be the Vice-President, if such number be a majority of the whole number of Electors appointed, and if no person have a majority, then from the two highest numbers on the list, the Senate shall choose the Vice-President; a quorum for the purpose shall consist of two-thirds of the whole number of Senators, and a majority of the whole number shall be necessary to a choice. But no person constitutionally ineligible to the office of President shall be eligible to that of Vice-President of the United States. *Superseded by section 3 of the 20th amendment.

AMENDMENT XIII

Passed by Congress January 31, 1865. Ratified December 6, 1865.

Note: A portion of Article IV, section 2, of the Constitution was superseded by the 13th amendment.

Section 1.

Neither slavery nor involuntary servitude, except as a punishment for crime whereof the party shall have been duly convicted, shall exist within the United States, or any place subject to their jurisdiction.

Section 2.

Congress shall have power to enforce this article by appropriate legislation.

AMENDMENT XIV

Passed by Congress June 13, 1866. Ratified July 9, 1868.

Note: Article I, section 2, of the Constitution was modified by section 2 of the 14th amendment.

Section 1.

All persons born or naturalized in the United States, and subject to the jurisdiction thereof, are citizens of the United States and of the State wherein they reside. No State shall make or enforce any law which shall abridge the privileges or immunities of citizens of the United States; nor shall any State deprive any person of life, liberty, or property, without due process of law; nor deny to any person within its jurisdiction the equal protection of the laws.

Section 2.

Representatives shall be apportioned among the several States according to their respective numbers, counting the whole number of persons in each State, excluding Indians not taxed. But when the right to vote at any election for the choice of electors for President and Vice-President of the United States, Representatives in Congress, the Executive and Judicial officers of a State, or the members of the Legislature thereof, is denied to any of the male inhabitants of such State, being twenty-one years of age,★ and citizens of the United States, or in any way abridged, except for participation in rebellion, or other crime, the basis of representation therein shall be reduced in the proportion which the number of such male citizens shall bear to the whole number of male citizens twenty-one years of age in such State.

Section 3.

No person shall be a Senator or Representative in Congress, or elector of President and Vice-President, or hold any office, civil or military, under the United States, or under any State, who, having previously taken an oath, as a member of Congress, or as an officer of the United States, or as a member of any State legislature, or as an executive or judicial officer of any State, to support the Constitution of the United States, shall have engaged in insurrection or rebellion against the same, or given aid or comfort to the enemies thereof. But Congress may by a vote of two-thirds of each House, remove such disability.

Section 4.

The validity of the public debt of the United States, authorized by law, including debts incurred for payment of pensions and bounties for services in suppressing insurrection or rebellion, shall not be questioned. But neither the United States nor any State shall assume or pay any debt or obligation incurred in aid of insurrection or rebellion against the United States, or any claim for the loss or emancipation of any slave; but all such debts, obligations and claims shall be held illegal and void.

Section 5.

The Congress shall have the power to enforce, by appropriate legislation, the provisions of this article.

*Changed by section 1 of the 26th amendment.

AMENDMENT XV

Passed by Congress February 26, 1869. Ratified February 3, 1870.

Section 1.

The right of citizens of the United States to vote shall not be denied or abridged by the United States or by any State on account of race, color, or previous condition of servitude--

Section 2.

The Congress shall have the power to enforce this article by appropriate legislation.

AMENDMENT XVI

Passed by Congress July 2, 1909. Ratified February 3, 1913.

Note: Article I, section 9, of the Constitution was modified by amendment 16.

The Congress shall have power to lay and collect taxes on incomes, from whatever source derived, without apportionment among the several States, and without regard to any census or enumeration.

AMENDMENT XVII

Passed by Congress May 13, 1912. Ratified April 8, 1913.

Note: Article I, section 3, of the Constitution was modified by the 17th amendment.

The Senate of the United States shall be composed of two Senators from each State, elected by the people thereof, for six years; and each Senator shall have one vote. The electors in each State shall have the qualifications requisite for electors of the most numerous branch of the State legislatures.

When vacancies happen in the representation of any State in the Senate, the executive authority of such State shall issue writs of election to fill such vacancies: Provided, That the legislature of any State may empower the executive thereof to make temporary appointments until the people fill the vacancies by election as the legislature may direct.

This amendment shall not be so construed as to affect the election or term of any Senator chosen before it becomes valid as part of the Constitution.

AMENDMENT XVIII

Passed by Congress December 18, 1917. Ratified January 16, 1919. Repealed by amendment 21.

Section 1.

After one year from the ratification of this article the manufacture, sale, or transportation of intoxicating liquors within, the importation thereof into, or the exportation thereof from the United States and all territory subject to the jurisdiction thereof for beverage purposes is hereby prohibited.

Section 2.

The Congress and the several States shall have concurrent power to enforce this article by appropriate legislation.

Section 3.

This article shall be inoperative unless it shall have been ratified as an amendment to the Constitution by the legislatures of the several States, as provided in the Constitution, within seven years from the date of the submission hereof to the States by the Congress.

AMENDMENT XIX

Passed by Congress June 4, 1919. Ratified August 18, 1920.

The right of citizens of the United States to vote shall not be denied or abridged by the United States or by any State on account of sex.

Congress shall have power to enforce this article by appropriate legislation.

AMENDMENT XX

Passed by Congress March 2, 1932. Ratified January 23, 1933.

Note: Article I, section 4, of the Constitution was modified by section 2 of this amendment. In addition, a portion of the 12th amendment was superseded by section 3.

Section 1.

The terms of the President and the Vice President shall end at noon on the 20th day of January, and the terms of Senators and Representatives at noon on the 3d day of January, of the years in which such terms would have ended if this article had not been ratified; and the terms of their successors shall then begin.

Section 2.

The Congress shall assemble at least once in every year, and such meeting shall begin at noon on the 3d day of January, unless they shall by law appoint a different day.

Section 3.

If, at the time fixed for the beginning of the term of the President, the President elect shall have died, the Vice President elect shall become President. If a President shall not have been chosen before the time fixed for the beginning of his term, or if the President elect shall have failed to qualify, then the Vice President elect shall act as President until a President shall have qualified; and the Congress may by law provide for the case wherein neither a President elect nor a Vice President elect shall have qualified, declaring who shall then act as President, or the manner in which one who is to act shall be selected, and such person shall act accordingly until a President or Vice President shall have qualified.

Section 4.

The Congress may by law provide for the case of the death of any of the persons from whom the House of Representatives may choose a President whenever the right of choice shall have devolved upon them, and for the case of the death of any of the persons from whom the Senate may choose a Vice President whenever the right of choice shall have devolved upon them.

Section 5.

Sections 1 and 2 shall take effect on the 15th day of October following the ratification of this article.

Section 6.

This article shall be inoperative unless it shall have been ratified as an amendment to the Constitution by the legislatures of three-fourths of the several States within seven years from the date of its submission.

AMENDMENT XXI

Passed by Congress February 20, 1933. Ratified December 5, 1933.

Section 1.

The eighteenth article of amendment to the Constitution of the United States is hereby repealed

Section 2.

The transportation or importation into any State, Territory, or possession of the United States for delivery or use therein of intoxicating liquors, in violation of the laws thereof, is hereby prohibited.

Section 3.

This article shall be inoperative unless it shall have been ratified as an amendment to the Constitution by conventions in the several States, as provided in the Constitution, within seven years from the date of the submission hereof to the States by the Congress.

AMENDMENT XXII

Passed by Congress March 21, 1947. Ratified February 27, 1951.

Section 1.

No person shall be elected to the office of the President more than twice, and no person who has held the office of President, or acted as President, for more than two years of a term to which some other person was elected President shall be elected to the office of the President more than once. But this Article shall not apply to any person holding the office of President when this Article was proposed by the Congress, and shall not prevent any person who may be holding the office of President, or acting as President, during the term within which this Article becomes operative from holding the office of President or acting as President during the remainder of such term.

Section 2.

This article shall be inoperative unless it shall have been ratified as an amendment to the Constitution by the legislatures of three-fourths of the several States within seven years from the date of its submission to the States by the Congress.

AMENDMENT XXIII

Passed by Congress June 16, 1960. Ratified March 29, 1961.

Section 1.

The District constituting the seat of Government of the United States shall appoint in such manner as the Congress may direct:

A number of electors of President and Vice President equal to the whole number of Senators and Representatives in Congress to which the District would be entitled if it were a State, but in no event more than the least populous State; they shall be in addition to those appointed by the States, but they shall be considered, for the purposes of the election of President and Vice President, to be electors appointed by a State; and they shall meet in the District and perform such duties as provided by the twelfth article of amendment.

Section 2.

The Congress shall have power to enforce this article by appropriate legislation.

AMENDMENT XXIV

Passed by Congress August 27, 1962. Ratified January 23, 1964.

Section 1.

The right of citizens of the United States to vote in any primary or other election for President or Vice President, for electors for President or Vice President, or for Senator or Representative in Congress, shall not be denied or abridged by the United States or any State by reason of failure to pay any poll tax or other tax.

Section 2.

The Congress shall have power to enforce this article by appropriate legislation.

AMENDMENT XXV

Passed by Congress July 6, 1965. Ratified February 10, 1967.

Note: Article II, section 1, of the Constitution was affected by the 25th amendment.

Section 1.

In case of the removal of the President from office or of his death or resignation, the Vice President shall become President.

Section 2.

Whenever there is a vacancy in the office of the Vice President, the President shall nominate a Vice President who shall take office upon confirmation by a majority vote of both Houses of Congress.

Section 3.

Whenever the President transmits to the President pro tempore of the Senate and the Speaker of the House of Representatives his written declaration that he is unable to discharge the powers and duties of his office, and until he transmits to them a written declaration to the contrary, such powers and duties shall be discharged by the Vice President as Acting President.

Section 4.

Whenever the Vice President and a majority of either the principal officers of the executive departments or of such other body as Congress may by law provide, transmit to the President pro tempore of the Senate and the Speaker of the House of Representatives their written declaration that the President is unable to discharge the powers and duties of his office, the Vice President shall immediately assume the powers and duties of the office as Acting President.

Thereafter, when the President transmits to the President pro tempore of the Senate and the Speaker of the House of Representatives his written declaration that no inability exists, he shall resume the powers and duties of his office unless the Vice President and a majority of either the principal officers of the executive department or of such other body as Congress may by law provide, transmit within four days to the President pro tempore of the Senate and the Speaker of the House of Representatives their written declaration that the President is unable to discharge the powers and duties of his office. Thereupon Congress shall decide the issue, assembling within forty-eight hours for that purpose if not in session. If the Congress, within twenty-one days after receipt of the latter written declaration, or, if Congress is not in session, within twenty-one days after Congress is required to assemble, determines by two-thirds vote of both Houses that the President is unable to discharge the powers and duties of his office, the Vice President shall continue to discharge the same as Acting President; otherwise, the President shall resume the powers and duties of his office.

AMENDMENT XXVI

Passed by Congress March 23, 1971. Ratified July 1, 1971.

Note: Amendment 14, section 2, of the Constitution was modified by section 1 of the 26th amendment.

Section 1.

The right of citizens of the United States, who are eighteen years of age or older, to vote shall not be denied or abridged by the United States or by any State on account of age.

Section 2.

The Congress shall have power to enforce this article by appropriate legislation.

AMENDMENT XXVII

Originally proposed Sept. 25, 1789. Ratified May 7, 1992.

No law, varying the compensation for the services of the Senators and Representatives, shall take effect, until an election of Representatives shall have intervened.

The Federalist, commonly referred to as the Federalist Papers, is a series of 85 essays written by Alexander Hamilton, John Jay, and James Madison between October 1787 and May 1788. The essays were published anonymously, under the pen name "Publius," in various New York state newspapers of the time.

The Federalist Papers were written and published to urge New Yorkers to ratify the proposed United States Constitution, which was drafted in Philadelphia in the summer of 1787. In lobbying for adoption of the Constitution over the existing Articles of Confederation, the essays explain particular provisions of the Constitution in detail. For this reason, and because Hamilton and Madison were each members of the

Constitutional Convention, the Federalist Papers are often used today to help interpret the intentions of those drafting the Constitution.

The Federalist Papers were published primarily in two New York state newspapers: *The New York Packet* and *The Independent journal.* They were reprinted in other newspapers in New York state and in several cities in other states. A bound edition, with revisions and corrections by Hamilton, was published in 1788 by printers J. and A. McLean. An edition published by printer Jacob Gideon in 1818, with revisions and corrections by Madison, was the first to identify each essay by its author's name. Because of its publishing history, the assignment of authorship, numbering, and exact wording may vary with different editions of *The Federalist.*

The electronic text of *The Federalist* used here was compiled for Project Gutenberg by scholars who drew on many available versions of the papers.

One printed edition of the text is *The Federalist,* edited by Jacob E. Cooke (Middletown, Conn., Wesleyan University Press, 1961). Cooke's introduction provides background information on the printing history of The Federalist; the information provided above comes in part from his work.

This web-friendly presentation of the original text of the Federalist Papers (also known as The Federalist) was obtained from the e-text archives of Project Gutenberg. Any irregularities with regard to grammar, syntax, spelling, or punctuation are as they exist in the original e-text archives.

TABLE OF CONTENTS

11.	The Utility of the Union in Respect to Commercial Relations and a Navy	Hamilton	For the *Independent Journal*	--
12.	The Utility of the Union in Respect to Revenue	Hamilton	From the *New York Packet*	Tuesday, November 27, 1787
13.	Advantage of the Union in Respect to Economy in Government	Hamilton	For the *Independent Journal*	--
14.	Objections to the Proposed Constitution from Extent of Territory Answered	Madison	From the *New York Packet*	Friday, November 30, 1787
15.	The Insufficiency of the Present Confederation to Preserve the Union	Hamilton	For the *Independent Journal*	--
16.	The Same Subject Continued: The Insufficiency of the Present Confederation to Preserve the Union	Hamilton	For the *Independent Journal*	Tuesday, December 4, 1787
17.	The Same Subject Continued: The Insufficiency of the Present Confederation to Preserve the Union	Hamilton	For the *Independent Journal*	--
18.	The Same Subject Continued: The Insufficiency of the Present Confederation to Preserve the Union	Hamilton and Madison	For the *Independent Journal*	--
19.	The Same Subject Continued: The Insufficiency of the Present Confederation to Preserve the Union	Hamilton and Madison	For the *Independent Journal*	--

20.	The Same Subject Continued: The Insufficiency of the Present Confederation to Preserve the Union	Hamilton and Madison	From the *New York Packet*	Tuesday, December 11, 1787
21.	Other Defects of the Present Confederation	Hamilton	For the *Independent Journal*	--
22.	The Same Subject Continued: Other Defects of the Present Confederation	Hamilton	From the *New York Packet*	Friday, December 14, 1787
23.	The Necessity of a Government as Energetic as the One Proposed to the Preservation of the Union.	Hamilton	From the *New York Packet*	Tuesday, December 17, 1787
24.	The Powers Necessary to the Common Defense Further Considered	Hamilton	For the *Independent Journal*	--
25.	The Same Subject Continued: The Powers Necessary to the Common Defense Further Considered	Hamilton	From the *New York Packet*	Friday, December 21, 1787
26.	The Idea of Restraining the Legislative Authority in Regard to the Common Defense Considered	Hamilton	For the *Independent Journal*	--
27.	The Same Subject Continued: The Idea of Restraining the Legislative Authority in Regard to the Common Defense Considered	Hamilton	From the *New York Packet*	Tuesday, December 25, 1787
28.	The Same Subject Continued: The Idea of Restraining the Legislative Authority in Regard to the Common Defense Considered	Hamilton	For the *Independent Journal*	--

29.	Concerning the Militia	Hamilton	From the *Daily Advertiser*	Thursday, January 10, 1788
30.	Concerning the General Power of Taxation	Hamilton	From the *New York Packet*	Friday, December 28, 1787
31.	The Same Subject Continued: Concerning the Power of Taxation	Hamilton	From the *New York Packet*	Tuesday, January 1, 1788
32.	The Same Subject Continued: Concerning the Power of Taxation	Hamilton	From the *Daily Advertiser*	Thursday, January 3, 1788
33.	The Same Subject Continued: Concerning the Power of Taxation	Hamilton	From the *Daily Advertiser*	Thursday, January 3, 1788
34.	The Same Subject Continued: Concerning the Power of Taxation	Hamilton	From the *New York Packet*	Friday, January 4, 1788
35.	The Same Subject Continued: Concerning the Power of Taxation	Hamilton	For the *Independent Journal*	--
36.	The Same Subject Continued: Concerning the Power of Taxation	Hamilton	From the *New York Packet*	Tuesday, January 8, 1788
37.	Concerning the Difficulties of the Convention in Devising a Proper Form of Government	Madison	From the *Daily Advertiser*	Friday, January 11, 1788
38.	Incoherence of the Objections to the New Plan Exposed	Madison	From the *New York Packet*	Tuesday, January 15, 1788
39.	Conformity of the Plan to Republican Principles	Madison	For the *Independent Journal*	--

50.	Periodic Appeals to the People Considered	Hamilton or Madison	From the *New York Packet*	Tuesday, February 5, 1788
51.	The Structure of the Government Must Furnish the Proper Checks and Balances Between the Different Departments	Hamilton or Madison	From the *New York Packet*	Friday, February 8, 1788
52.	The House of Representatives	Hamilton or Madison	From the *New York Packet*	Friday, February 8, 1788
53.	The Same Subject Continued: The House of Representatives	Hamilton or Madison	From the *New York Packet*	Tuesday, February 12, 1788
54.	The Apportionment of Members Among States	Hamilton or Madison	From the *New York Packet*	Tuesday, February 12, 1788
55.	The Total Number of the House of Representatives	Hamilton or Madison	From the *New York Packet*	Friday, February 15, 1788
56.	The Same Subject Continued: The Total Number of the House of Representatives	Hamilton or Madison	From the *New York Packet*	Tuesday, February 19, 1788
57.	The Alleged Tendency of the Plan to Elevate the Few at the Expense of the Many Considered in Connection with Representation	Hamilton or Madison	friend	Tuesday, February 19, 1788
58.	Objection that the Number of Members Will Not Be Augmented as the Progress of Population Demands Considered	Madison	--	--

59.	Concerning the Power of Congress to Regulate the Election of Members	Hamilton	From the *New York Packet*	Friday, February 22, 1788
60.	The Same Subject Continued: Concerning the Power of Congress to Regulate the Election of Members	Hamilton	From the *New York Packet*	Tuesday, February 26, 1788
61.	The Same Subject Continued: Concerning the Power of Congress to Regulate the Election of Members	Hamilton	From the *New York Packet*	Tuesday, February 26, 1788
62.	The Senate	Hamilton or Madison	For the *Independent Journal*	--
63.	The Senate Continued	Hamilton or Madison	For the *Independent Journal*	--
64.	The Powers of the Senate	Jay	From the *New York Packet*	Friday, March 7, 1788
65.	The Powers of the Senate Continued	Hamilton	From the *New York Packet*	Friday, March 7, 1788
66.	Objections to the Power of the Senate To Set as a Court for Impeachments Further Considered	Hamilton	From the *New York Packet*	Tuesday, March 11, 1788
67.	The Executive Department	Hamilton	From the *New York Packet*	Tuesday, March 11, 1788
68.	The Mode of Electing the President	Hamilton	From the *New York Packet*	Friday, March 14, 1788
69.	The Real Character of the Executive	Hamilton	From the *New York Packet*	Friday, March 14, 1788

70.	The Executive Department Further Considered	Hamilton	From the *New York Packet*	Friday, March 14, 1788
71.	The Duration in Office of the Executive	Hamilton	From the *New York Packet*	Tuesday, March 18, 1788
72.	The Same Subject Continued, and Re-Eligibility of the Executive Considered	Hamilton	From the *New York Packet*	Friday, March 21, 1788
73.	The Provision for Support of the Executive, and the Veto Power	Hamilton	From the *New York Packet*	Friday, March 21, 1788
74.	The Command of the Military and Naval Forces, and the Pardoning Power of the Executive	Hamilton	From the *New York Packet*	Tuesday, March 25, 1788
75.	The Treaty Making Power of the Executive	Hamilton	For the *Independent Journal*	--
76.	The Appointing Power of the Executive	Hamilton	From the *New York Packet*	Tuesday, April 1, 1788
77.	The Appointing Power Continued and Other Powers of the Executive Considered	Hamilton	From the *New York Packet*	Friday, April 4, 1788
78.	The Judiciary Department	Hamilton	From McLEAN's Edition, New York	--
79.	The Judiciary Continued	Hamilton	From McLEAN's Edition, New York	--
80.	The Powers of the Judiciary	Hamilton	From McLEAN's Edition, New York	--

So as I conclude my book.

I also enter into the next chapter of my life, the chapter that does not include going to a job every day, I intend to spend as much time as possible with my children and grandchildren (and if I live long enough) my Great grandchildren, I also want to make a difference in my Community, what form this will take (as of now I do not know) thru a lot of reflecting on the past and asking God in prayer to let me know what he wants me to do with my remaining years, everything leads me to the same conclusion. I need to tell people about the journey I have made in my life and how God protected me and nudged me to where he wanted me to go in life and of all the miracles that God used to get me there, I pray that when I get to Heaven Jesus will be happy with how I spent my remaining years on this Earth. Thank you and may God bless you.

ABOUT THE AUTHOR

He has no previous experience writing a book. He has resisted writing this book for many years. God has nudged the Author to share what God has done for him . This book is his attempt to do just that. The Author was born in 1961, born into a poor family in rural Illinois. He struggled to graduate high school and did not pursue Higher education. He worked most of his adult life in retail. Most of his retail experience was being the Store Manager of Walmart Stores, starting with a very small store doing 7 Million dollars of sales a year, ending with a Walmart Supercenter doing over 100 Million dollars of sales a year. The Author managed this store, located in Columbia, Tennessee, for over 22 years. The Author has been married for over 37 years. He and his wife, Ramona, have 4 children and 7 grandchildren, with another on the way

   The Author accepted Jesus as his Savior on 12-15-1996 at the age of 35. That miraculous event has totally changed his life.

Printed in the United States
by Baker & Taylor Publisher Services